Palgrave Studies in Science and Popular Culture

Series Editor
Sherryl Vint
Department of English
University of California
Riverside, CA, USA

This book series seeks to publish ground-breaking research exploring the productive intersection of science and the cultural imagination. Science is at the centre of daily experience in twenty-first century life and this has defined moments of intense technological change, such as the Space Race of the 1950s and our very own era of synthetic biology. Conceived in dialogue with the field of Science and Technology Studies (STS), this series will carve out a larger place for the contribution of humanities to these fields. The practice of science is shaped by the cultural context in which it occurs and cultural differences are now key to understanding the ways that scientific practice is enmeshed in global issues of equity and social justice. We seek proposals dealing with any aspect of science in popular culture in any genre. We understand popular culture as both a textual and material practice, and thus welcome manuscripts dealing with representations of science in popular culture and those addressing the role of the cultural imagination in material encounters with science. How science is imagined and what meanings are attached to these imaginaries will be the major focus of this series. We encourage proposals from a wide range of historical and cultural perspectives.

Alicia Castillo Villanueva • Angelos Bollas
Editors

HIV/AIDS in Memory, Culture and Society

palgrave
macmillan

Editors
Alicia Castillo Villanueva
SALIS
Dublin City University
Dublin, Ireland

Angelos Bollas
Department of Sociology
Maynooth University
Maynooth, Ireland

ISSN 2731-4359 ISSN 2731-4367 (electronic)
Palgrave Studies in Science and Popular Culture
ISBN 978-3-031-59698-8 ISBN 978-3-031-59699-5 (eBook)
https://doi.org/10.1007/978-3-031-59699-5

Cover illustration: KATERYNA KON/SCIENCE PHOTO LIBRARY / Getty Images

This Palgrave Macmillan imprint is published by the registered company Springer Nature Switzerland AG.
The registered company address is: Gewerbestrasse 11, 6330 Cham, Switzerland

Paper in this product is recyclable.

To those affected by HIV/AIDS in the past, the present, and the future
To Willie, Guillermo and David. To my parents
To Apostolos

Acknowledgements

We would like to extend our thanks to everyone who has contributed to making this book possible. First, we would like to thank our editor Camille Davis for all the support she has given us on this long journey. Additionally, we would like to express our gratitude to Karthika Devi Ravikumar and the production team at Palgrave Macmillan. We are deeply grateful to all the contributors for their knowledge, effort, and commitment to this project. Their work ethic has made this book possible. Our sincere gratitude to the Faculty of Humanities and Social Sciences for the financial support provided for the completion of this book and other events related to the topic such as the HIV/AIDS: Then and Now conference held in 2019 at Dublin City University, Ireland. Many thanks to all peer-reviewers for giving us their time and exceptional work. Their valuable recommendations and expertise have contributed to expanding our knowledge and the exchange of ideas. We cannot forget Dr Sarah Meehan O'Callaghan and Jeremy Murphy from JM Agency for their meticulous copy-editing work. Finally, many thanks to our families and friends who have supported us unconditionally, as always.

We hope that this book contributes to recovering silenced voices of the past and to giving voice to those who are still not heard so that they can become part of the collective and transcultural memory of HIV/AIDS. Their narratives not only represent a form of resistance, but also a way of engaging in a language of social justice.

Contents

Notes on Contributors

Angelos Bollas is an Assistant Lecturer in the Department of Sociology at Maynooth University. His research focuses on masculinities and sexuality studies from sociological and cultural studies perspectives. He writes about societal discrimination in relation to sexuality, cultural representations of masculinities, expressions of masculinities which challenge normative understandings of gender and sexuality, as well as pedagogical considerations around inclusion and diversity. His work appears in peer-reviewed journals such as the *Journal of Homosexuality*, *Journal of Bisexuality*, and *Sexuality & Culture*. He is the author of *Contemporary Irish Masculinities* (Routledge), *Sexualised Governmentalities* (Springer), and *Fashionable Queerness* (Emerald).

Alicia Castillo Villanueva is an Assistant Professor in Hispanic Studies, Gender and Sexuality at the School of Applied Language and Intercultural Studies (SALIS) in Dublin City University. She lectures and researches on the field of Feminist studies with a focus on the social and cultural representations of different forms of gender-based violence, conflict, and memory. Alicia has published widely in top international journals such as *PLoS One*, the *Spanish Journal of Sociology*, *Perspectives*, or *Bulletin of Spanish Studies.* In addition, she explores the intersection of translation, conflict, and memory and is the co-author of *New Approaches to Translation, Conflict and Memory* (Palgrave Macmillan).

Ellie Marley was awarded a PhD from the School of Nursing, Psychotherapy and Community Health in Dublin City University in 2022. Her thesis adopted narrative inquiry to explore how shame features in the lives of women living with HIV in Ireland. Ellie currently works with the National Care Experience Programme at Health Information and Quality Authority (HIQA), a joint initiative between HIQA, the Department for Health, and the Health Service Executive, working to improve the quality of care delivered across Ireland. Ellie's research interest includes employing qualitative methods to explore HIV shame and stigma and researching with marginalised and seldom heard voices.

Elizabeth Mills is a Senior Lecturer in the Departments of Anthropology and International Development at the University of Sussex. Originally from South Africa, she has engaged with policy and conducted research around the world on HIV, gender, health, medicine, queer kinship, and human rights. Using visual anthropological approaches—including film, photography, body mapping, and digital mapping—her ethnographic research has explored women's embodied accounts of HIV and AIDS biomedicines in South Africa and Brazil. This ethnography reflects two decades of research in South Africa and elsewhere (including Sierra Leone and Brazil), with related publications on stigma, the politics of biomedicine, traditional healing, gender, violence, and masculinities.

David O'Mullane is a doctoral scholar at Dublin City University. His PhD, *The Art of Cruising: Queer Sexual Politics and Contemporary Visual Culture*, explores how public sex is denigrated, politicised, or idealised within contemporary queer culture and theory. Beyond his PhD, his research interests extend to visual culture's intersection with queer theory, embodiment, and artivism. David co-organized the 2023 SEX Pan!cs International Conference and co-founded *Cruising*, a magazine publication exploring sexual subcultures, with artist and academic Matt Ryalls.

Denise Proudfoot is an Assistant Professor at School of Nursing, Psychotherapy and Community Health in DCU. She is a nurse academic with both clinical and research experience in the area of HIV sexual and mental health. She was awarded a Doctorate in Health from University of Bath, UK and her thesis was a narrative study about mothering while HIV positive. She currently lectures on a variety of topics including mental health, sexual health, and sexuality in nursing. As a researcher her interests are in the area of HIV and amp; inclusion health with a particular focus on gender.

Mirta Suquet is an Assistant Professor of Spanish Studies in the Department of Languages, Literatures and Cultures at Susquehanna University. Her research delves into the representation of mental illness, disabilities, and diseases in literature, cinema, and visual arts. She explores notions of contagion, pollution, and abjection related to gender, race, ethnicity, or sexual orientation, along with strategies of resistance and subversion employed by writers and artists. Suquet's work includes the study of authors such as Reinaldo Arenas and Severo Sarduy. She recently contributed to Revista Tesis with '*Cuba in Quarantine: Images of Precarity and Vulnerability during the COVID Pandemic in 2023*'.

Janey Umback BA (Hons) is a PhD candidate in the department of Internet Studies at Curtin University, Western Australia. Her PhD project is an examination of intimate publics within both Harry Styles and BTS ARMY fan communities. She is a research student at the Influencer Ethnography Research Lab (IERLab), and an associate student of the Korea Research Centre (KRC). Janey has previously published work relating to fan communities associated with Harry Styles.

List of Figures

CHAPTER 1

Viral Echoes: Revisiting the Cultural Memory of HIV/AIDS

Alicia Castillo Villanueva and Angelos Bollas

1.1 Introduction

This book is a collection of chapters that examines different cultural and social representations of HIV/AIDS from the contemporary perspective of memory. The volume presents different facets of the existing dialogue between HIV/AIDS and cultural memory from a plurality of disciplines and perspectives, including HIV/AIDS studies, artivism, media studies, medical humanities, ethnography studies, and queer studies. This volume explores the scope of memory, culture, and society in re-examining experiences of HIV/AIDS and the importance of recording, writing, and performing in preserving the memories of the AIDS pandemic and personal views and understanding. By examining these representations, this edited

A. Castillo Villanueva (✉)
SALIS, Dublin City University, Dublin, Ireland
e-mail: Alicia.castillovillanueva@dcu.ie

A. Bollas
Department of Sociology, Maynooth University, Maynooth, Ireland
e-mail: angelos.bollas@mu.ie

A. Castillo Villanueva, A. Bollas (eds.), *HIV/AIDS in Memory, Culture and Society*, Palgrave Studies in Science and Popular Culture, https://doi.org/10.1007/978-3-031-59699-5_1

book reflects on how HIV/AIDS has been portrayed in diverse socio-cultural constituencies. In the chapters that follow, authors consider the challenges in representing and disseminating new discourses of the pandemic in specific contexts, which allows for an intergenerational and trans-cultural dialogue and analysis of the landscape of HIV/AIDS as well as other representations of illness.

Since the publication of the first scientific report on AIDS, the Morbidity and Mortality Weekly Report from the United States Centres for Diseases Control (CDC 1981), medical advances have occurred that have changed the paradigm of the disease at different levels in contemporary societies. The widespread designation of HIV/AIDS as 'the gay disease' caused the silence and inaction of many political leaders and the media. In a recent book, *New York Times* journalist Adam Nagourney (2023) reveals how the newspaper did not provide sufficient coverage of the disease for years due to the homophobic prejudice of its assigned editor, Abe Rosenthal. The slow and inadequate response in the United States by President Ronald Reagan's administration had serious consequences on the spread of the virus and the tide of deaths that could have been slowed and unnecessary suffering prevented (Shilts 2011). At the first White House press conference on AIDS in 1982, the president's aides made anti-gay jibes while noting that about a third of reported cases were fatal (Beyrer 2021). The slow and ruthless response by governments was due to the association of the virus with homosexuality and bisexuality. In the UK, the Thatcher government was also slow to respond, and it was not until 1986 that an HIV/AIDS public health and education policy was formalised even though Nicholas Eden, 2nd Lord of Avon, Under Secretary of the Environment, died from AIDS in 1985. We must not forget that Thatcher's government also adopted homophobic laws such as Section 28 of the Local Government Act, which banned the 'promotion of homosexuality' in schools. The law was passed in 1988, in the aftermath of the new public awareness of AIDS in which gay people were linked with amorality and disease (Stacey 1991; Thomson 1993; Moran 2001). Perhaps the most controversial and infamous response in the history of HIV/AIDS was that of Thabo Mbeki's government in South Africa. From the first death from AIDS in 1981 until a decade later, the government paid little attention to a pandemic that affected homosexual men, haemophiliacs, and foreign African mineworkers (Simelela et al. 2015). Lack of information, together with other demands from the new government to dismantle apartheid structures, meant that the HIV pandemic was relegated to the background in 1994 under Mandela's government. Since the late 1990s, the Mbeki government has been defined by denying that AIDS was caused by a virus. As a result of the denialist response, an estimated 330,000 people died due to the lack of provision of antiretroviral therapy (ART) (Chigwedere et al. 2008). China did not declare AIDS a reportable disease until 1991 but banned all HIV-infected foreigners from entering the country in 1988 (He and Detels 2005). With the appearance of the first cases of AIDS in 1985, a system of mandatory confinement for all those affected began in Cuba, which prevailed until 1993. The negative responses of governments only intensified stigma, discrimination, and even collective denial of the pandemic at a social level.

Beyrer (2021) points out how the inadequate and slow response and the absence of any effective therapy generated a fierce wave of activism. The involvement of the gay community was essential for governments to launch preventive education programmes. Various organisations established activities that included voluntary action, peer education, care, and public activism. Many American-born organisations, such as Gay Men's Health Crisis (GMHC) in New York and the Kaposi Foundation for Sarcoma Research and Education in San Francisco (later renamed the San Francisco AIDS Foundation), exerted a significant influence throughout the Western world (Robinson 2014). Beyrer (2021) recounts how media-savvy activists, passionate and galvanised by seeing friends and lovers die, faced different insensitive, hostile, and AIDS-denial governments. Activists educated themselves on everything from trial designs to antiviral mechanisms and changed the way medical research has been conducted ever since. Debates and discourses linking HIV/AIDS with gay men and drug addiction led to the rise of rampant homophobia and stigmatisation that would limit crucial early responses to its spread.

It would be impossible to mention in this introduction all the associations and activists who around the world have contributed and continue to contribute to the cause of eradicating HIV/AIDS and ensuring that people have access to treatments worldwide. The 15 years that elapsed between the emergence of AIDS and the development of effective antiretroviral therapy (ART) in 1996 were devastating (Beyrer 2021). New therapies changed the reality of the pandemic, and while deaths decreased in high-income countries, middle- and low-income countries saw an increase in lives lost between the period from 1993 to 2003 due to the high cost of treatments. The Joint United Nations Programme on HIV/AIDS (UNAIDS), launched in 1994, aimed to unite the world against AIDS and lead and inspire countries to ensure access to care, treatment, and prevention for all. At the turn of the millennium, unequal access to life-saving antiviral medications caused civil society groups such as the Treatment Action Campaign (TAC) in South Africa to mobilise (Bekker 2023). The Global Fund to Fight AIDS, Tuberculosis and Malaria founded in 2002 (the world's largest funder of AIDS, tuberculosis and malaria prevention, treatment, and care programmes), together with the President's Emergency Plan for Relief of AIDS (PEPFAR) created in 2003 by George W. Bush, led to the investment of more than 100 billion dollars in the global response to HIV/AIDS, saving more than 25 million lives and helping to prevent and control the pandemic—all this substantially strengthening global economic security (Bekker 2023). Forty years since the identification of HIV/AIDS, infections and deaths continue despite the availability of treatment in regions with high incidence. HIV deaths continue to occur in Africa and East Asia, with rates increasing in regions of the Middle East, parts of North and West Africa, Central Asia, and Eastern Europe (UNAIDS 2023). UNAIDS' objectives 95-95-95 for 2025 are, on the one hand, to reduce punitive laws and policies, discrimination and stigma, and gender inequality and violence to below 10%. On the other hand, the organisation aims to increase access to treatment and testing, sexual and reproductive health services, and the elimination of vertical transmission to 95%. The Sustainable Development Goal (SDG) 3.3 expects to end AIDS as a public health threat by 2030.

One of the most important medical innovations in relation to the elimination of transmission is PrEP. PrEP, or pre-exposure prophylaxis, is a medication used to prevent HIV infection. It is taken daily and has been shown to be highly effective in preventing HIV transmission when used consistently (Spieldenner 2016). PrEP is typically prescribed for individuals who are HIV-negative but have a high risk of HIV infection, such as those who have HIV-positive partners, engage in high-risk sexual behaviour, or have a history of sexually transmitted infections (Karris et al. 2014). PrEP was first introduced in 2012 when the US Food and Drug Administration (FDA) approved the use of tenofovir disoproxil fumarate (TDF) as a daily oral medication to reduce the risk of HIV infection in adults and adolescents (Calabrese et al. 2019). In 2018, the FDA approved the use of emtricitabine/tenofovir alafenamide (F/TAF) as a daily oral medication for PrEP in adults and adolescents (Calabrese et al. 2019). Today, PrEP is widely used in the United States and other countries, with millions of people using it to protect themselves from HIV infection.

According to the Centers for Disease Control and Prevention (CDC), the number of people using PrEP in the United States increased from 100,000 in 2015 to 1.2 million in 2020 (Jackson et al. 2023). The CDC also reports that PrEP use has been associated with a 20% reduction in HIV transmission among gay and bisexual men and a 30% reduction in HIV transmission among transgender women (Grimshaw et al. 2021). In the Global South, PrEP has been introduced and adopted in various countries, with varying levels of success. According to the World Health Organisation (WHO), there were about 1.6 million people across the world who received oral PrEP at least once in 2021, with nearly 1 million of these being in eastern and southern Africa (HIV/AIDS (UNAIDS) 2022). In 2021, 144 countries reported that they had adopted the WHO recommendations on oral PrEP in national guidelines, with a further 14 countries reporting that they plan to adopt the recommendations in the next 2 years (HIV/AIDS (UNAIDS) 2022). However, there are still substantial gaps in the availability of PrEP, particularly in countries where it is not yet widely available or accessible (HIV/AIDS (UNAIDS) n.d.). For example, in South Africa, the overall level of PrEP awareness was 18.8%, but only 1.7% of participants had used PrEP, 7.5% had seen it, and 4.8% knew how much it cost (Adeniyi and Ter Goon 2019). This low awareness and use of PrEP in high HIV and sexual violence prevalence settings is a barrier to its use in the Global South (Ajayi et al. 2019).

1.2 The Memory of HIV/AIDS

In 2021, the 40th anniversary of HIV/AIDS was commemorated. Different organisations dedicated to eradicating the virus in the medical world, the cultural world, and the media, among others, reflected on the progress made and remembered those who died due to HIV/AIDS. The collective memory of HIV/AIDS is made up of individual memories that are shared through different forms and media, including debates, biographies, commemorations in public spaces, identity politics, oral history, and the culture of bearing witness. Maurice Halbwachs points out how the memory of events needs to be supported by a group that was involved, or that suffered the consequences of an event, that witnessed or received the oral accounts of the first actors or spectators (1992). The author also points out that the memory of a society extends until the groups are able to remember and dies when the members that make up the group disappear. But memory transforms and is dynamic; the groups change, but the memory continues and the interpretation of the past changes according to the transformations of the social frameworks in each present. Remembering means reconstructing the past in the present but also the emotions and affections associated with that past. Our volume focuses on the cultural memory of HIV/AIDS through different socio-cultural representations that come from oral voices collected from everyday interactions, but also from voices collected in other mediums such as literature, television, the media, and artworks. Although each society establishes its own way of relating to its past due to different customs, thoughts, policies, etc., the memory of HIV/AIDS must be conceived as 'travelling memory' and, therefore, as transcultural memory. Theories on cross-cultural memory arise due to a change in approach that assumes that memory is subject to a domestic frame of reference, that is, that of a limited nation-state. The frameworks of the recent so-called transcultural turn (Bond and Rapson 2014) take as reference the complexity of culture in a world characterised by processes of globalisation, transnational connections, and the break with notions of national or domestic memories (Brunow 2015). As a result, the theories proposed by Pierre Nora (1989) on *lieux de mémoire*, or sites of memory, are advanced in this volume. The frameworks of the recent so-called transcultural turn (Bond and Rapson 2014) take as reference the complexity of culture in a world characterised by processes of globalisation, transnational connections, and the break with notions of national or domestic memories (Brunow 2015). Astrid Erll formulates the concept of transculturality in memory studies as mnemonic processes that develop 'across and beyond cultures', that is, through and beyond cultures, which transcends the borders of traditional cultural memory studies (Erll 2011, 9). Bounded notions of nation-state cultures give way to more complex concepts of shared places of memory that have emerged because of trade, war, and migration exchanges, as well as colonial and postcolonial relations. Added to this, different social classes, generations, ethnicities, and subcultures that intersect within a nation, but also beyond it, must be considered, generating transnational networks of memory through cultural exchange (8). The author conceives transcultural memory as a dynamic entity that continually travels through different 'dimensions of movement' that she classifies as 'carriers, media, contents, forms and practices of memory', which are in continuous transformation through time and space and social, linguistic, and political borders (11). To stay alive and present, memory must travel and impact individual minds and social constructs. The continuous exchange of information between individuals through the dimensions of movement is fundamental for the formation of cross-cultural memory that is characterised as itinerant and dynamic (Erll 2011, 12). We must consider individuals who share images and collective narratives of the past as *carriers of memory*. Since the 1980s, many artists, writers, and directors, either directly affected by the virus or for ethical reasons, embarked on projects which offered a critical viewpoint. In so doing, their intentions were to raise social awareness and give agency to those affected by HIV/AIDS at the crossroads between the political and the poetic. Different mnemonic ritual practices have been carried out to remember and commemorate those affected by HIV/AIDS. An example of this is the NAMES project and the AIDS Memorial Quilt, which since 1987 has been expanded with the names of those who have perished due to HIV/AIDS. Throughout 1989, more than 20 countries held similar commemorations based on this project. From this project, others have been created, such as Call My Name in 2013, which focuses on the black community with HIV/AIDS and the public health crisis that still exists today. The programme aimed to raise awareness about the effect that persistent stigma and prejudice have on the black community.[1]

The creation of national memorials in public spaces in cities and in parks serves as places of memory in which ceremonies are held to commemorate and remember those affected by HIV/AIDS. Such mnemonic practices are adopted and travel across the world. Memorials to those who died are displayed in cities including Amsterdam, Auckland, Barcelona, Berlin, Brighton, Buenos Aires, Cape Town, Dublin, Edinburgh, Hong Kong, Johannesburg, Kiev, LA, Madrid, Manchester, Melbourne, Montreal, Moscow, Munich, NYC, Paris, San Francisco, San Salvador, Sydney, Toronto, Vienna, and Zurich. The Embraced Loop, the latest national memorial to 'remember and celebrate the lives of all those affected by HIV and AIDS', was unveiled in Phoenix Park in Dublin in December 2023.[2] London, in contrast to most other major cities, does not yet have a UKHIV/AIDS memorial, but funding to build one was announced on World AIDS Day in 2023.[3]

[1] More information about the history of the NAMES project and the Quilt can be found in the National AIDS Memorial website: https://www.aidsmemorial.org/quilt-history

[2] More information about the monument can be found at https://www.independent.ie/irish-news/phoenix-park-monument-to-those-affected-by-hiv-and-aids-unveiled/a10497827.html

[3] https://www.bbc.com/news/uk-england-london-67590449

The domain of Media, according to Erll (2011), constitutes in different ways and is a key dimension in how memory travels and is disseminated. Mnemonic content travels through media history in different forms, such as oral, written, and print. Also in the forms of films, documentaries, and the internet. Information transcription from one medium to another, or its 'travel' over time and technologies, has been researched under the umbrella of 'remediation' (Erll 2011; Brunow 2015). From 'remediation', the contents of cultural memory in the forms of images and narratives are created and shared, and their circulation causes the memories to be (re)actualised. In this sense, the incessant journey of content between the media and minds is in continuous reinterpretation and contestation, which causes the 'make of memory' (Erll 2011). Furthermore, this journey allows for the creation of continuity between the past and the present. It is crucial to bear in mind that 'memory in culture' is a multifaceted process that extends much beyond 'remembrance', let alone national memory. As Erll alerts us in her work, it implies knowledge, repertoires of stories and scripts, implicit memory, bodily elements like habitus, and—along with memory—forgetting. We have innumerable recollections of HIV/AIDS activism and resistance, hardship and victories; nevertheless, as the chapters in this book demonstrate, many others have been lost, silenced, and censored. But movements between borders are also subject to contingencies such as those of a linguistic nature and we must consider the key role of translation in the circulation of memories across borders (Pintado Gutiérrez and Castillo Villanueva 2019). Ultimately, memories that travel and circulate in different contexts aim to participate in a language that promotes social justice and the restoration of harm.

1.3 The Cultural Memory of HIV/AIDS

Homophobia and stigmatisation caused a widespread rejection and lack of interest towards the cultural representations of the pandemic in the first decade of the virus identification. Yet, soon afterwards, the medical progress which occurred since the development of antiretroviral therapy (ART) changed the lives of those affected by HIV/AIDS, shifting from *dying from it* to *living with it*. This new context gave rise to a general silence and lack of representation in some societies based on the wrong idea that HIV/AIDS could be cured, therefore ignoring the extension and consequences of the pandemic. As some of the chapters of this collection demonstrate, the 2010s brought about an increased interest in HIV/AIDS, which is recorded in a number of cultural products offering a nuanced view of the HIV/AIDS crisis and its continuing impact on society and which contribute to the ongoing dialogue about HIV/AIDS, blending historical context with contemporary insights.

The Love Positive Women project, established in 2013 by Visual AIDS artist member Jessica Whitbread, is a heartfelt initiative that intersects art, activism, and support for HIV-positive women. Partnering with MoMA PS1 in 2024, the project involves creating Valentine's Day cards on handmade paper by artists, activists, and HIV-positive women. This international series leverages Valentine's Day to foster acts of love and care for women living with HIV. The project addresses the isolation, stigma, and specific challenges faced by these women, with over 3500 cards distributed since 2015 to build community and empower them. Notable TV series and films on the topic of HIV/AIDS include: *Pose* (2018–2021), a groundbreaking TV series that depicts life in the 1980s for queer and trans people of colour in New York City, highlighting the impact of HIV during that era; *It's A Sin* (2021), a hit miniseries which explores the AIDS crisis in London during the 1980s and early 1990s, is praised for its raw portrayal of the pandemic's emotional impact; *United in Anger: A History of ACT UP* (2012), a documentary focusing on the AIDS activist movement from the perspective of those directly involved in fighting the pandemic; *How to Survive a Plague* (2012), a documentary which follows the origins of ACT UP and TAG, two activist organisations that transformed AIDS from a death sentence into a manageable condition; *How to Tell a Secret* (2023), a film which employs a blend of documentary and performance, utilising genre-blurring storytelling techniques to explore what it means to be HIV-positive in Ireland; and most recently *Fellow Travellers* (2023), a television miniseries, adapted from Thomas Mallon's 2007 novel, focusing on the enduring romantic relationship between two men during the peak of McCarthyism in the 1950s and spanning several decades.

In literature, *Tell the Wolves I'm Home* by Carol Rifka Brunt is a 2012 novel set in the 1980s. It tells the story of 14-year-old June Elbus, who mourns the loss of her uncle Finn, a beloved painter who dies of AIDS. June discovers Finn's secret friend, Toby, and together they explore their grief and the hidden parts of Finn's life, leading June to a deeper understanding of love, loss, and acceptance. *The Great Believers* by Rebecca Makkai, published in 2018, is a novel that intertwines two narratives set in different times. One part of the story is set in 1980s Chicago and focuses on the AIDS pandemic, portraying the impact on the gay community through the eyes of Yale Tishman and his friends. The other narrative takes place in 2015 Paris, following Fiona, the sister of one of Yale's friends who died from AIDS, as she searches for her estranged daughter. The novel explores themes of loss, memory, and the endurance of love amidst tragedy. *Funeral Diva* by Pamela Sneed, published in 2020, is a powerful collection of essays and poetry that combines personal narrative, political commentary, and cultural critique. Sneed reflects on her experiences as a black lesbian artist and activist, offering insights into issues of race, gender, and sexuality. The book provides a poignant account of the AIDS crisis and its impact on the LGBTQ+ community, as well as exploring themes of grief, survival, and resistance. *Funeral Diva* is both a memoir and a tribute to the lost and marginalised voices of the AIDS era.

Out of the Shadows: Reimagining Gay Men's Lives by Walt Odets is a 2020 reflective exploration of the lives and identities of gay men. The book examines the complexities faced by gay men in America, discussing the challenges of self-acceptance and the lasting impact of the AIDS pandemic. Odets, a clinical psychologist, draws from his experiences and patient stories to examine how early-life stigma and a lack of self-acceptance can affect gay men's lives. The work is an insightful blend of social commentary, memoir, and therapeutic analysis, aimed at helping gay men overcome trauma and isolation to live authentically and fulfillingly. *To Make the Wounded Whole: The African American Struggle Against HIV/AIDS* by Dan Royles, published in 2020, is a comprehensive exploration of the African American community's response to the HIV/AIDS pandemic. The book highlights the grassroots activism and community mobilisation that played a crucial role in addressing the crisis within the African American population. It sheds light on the intersection of race, health, and politics and chronicles the efforts of activists to combat both the disease and the underlying social and political challenges exacerbating its impact on the community. *All the Young Men* by Ruth Coker Burks, published in 2021, is a memoir that recounts Burks' experience as a young woman caring for men with AIDS in the 1980s in Arkansas. She steps into the role of a caregiver and advocate at a time when AIDS was heavily stigmatised and misunderstood. The book details her journey of compassion and activism as she helps these men in their final days, often being their only support in the face of societal and familial rejection. The memoir is a powerful story of empathy, resilience, and the human spirit in the face of a devastating pandemic.

Another Dimension of Us by Mike Albo is a 2023 science fiction novel blending elements of teen romance and astral travel. Set in 1986 and 2044, it follows Tommy Gaye, who harbours feelings for his best friend Renaldo during the AIDS crisis, and Pris Devrees, a student in 2044, navigating a world affected by a mysterious virus. The AIDS crisis of the 1980s is a significant backdrop to the story, particularly in the narrative set in 1986. The character Renaldo Calabasas, a talented writer, navigates the height of the AIDS crisis and the prevalent homophobia of that era. The impact of AIDS on the characters and their community is a critical element of the story/narrative reflecting the fear and stigma associated with the disease during that period. *Christodora* by Tim Murphy is a 2016 novel set in New York City, spanning several decades from the 1980s to the near future. It revolves around the residents of the Christodora, an apartment building in the East Village. The narrative weaves through the lives of various characters deeply affected by the AIDS pandemic, exploring themes of activism, addiction, family, and the impact of HIV/AIDS on the gay community. The story examines the personal and political ramifications of the crisis, showcasing the resilience and interconnectedness of its characters. *My Dead Book* by Nate Lippens is a 2022 novella that weaves together a series of vignettes and fragments. It follows the introspective journey of a queer man approaching his fiftieth birthday, haunted by memories of friends lost to the AIDS pandemic, his past as a sex worker, and reflections on survival and ageing in the queer community. The narrative captures the intimate, often painful, realities of dealing with trauma, loss, and identity, set against the backdrop of societal challenges faced by the LGBTQ community. *Living and Loving in the Age of AIDS* by Derek Frost is a 2021 memoir that narrates the story of Derek and his husband J, set against the backdrop of the AIDS pandemic. The book explores their lives filled with adventure and creativity, abruptly impacted by the arrival of AIDS. It recounts J's diagnosis with HIV, leading to a personal crisis amidst global stigma and fear. The memoir describes their journey of survival, spiritual reflection, and the creation of AIDS Ark, a charity saving the lives of HIV-positive individuals.

The literature related to the representation of HIV/AIDS through cultural and social debates is still a field in its infancy. The recent interest in recovering the cultural memory of HIV/AIDS is reflected in a small number of new publications, and for that reason, this book will be an addition to those already published on HIV/AIDS and its memory and legacy. As scholars in the field, we believe that this area will grow rapidly in the coming years as there is still a lack of studies that focus on the cultural memory of the pandemic in many countries, which are not included in this volume.

Current research shows a growing interest in revisiting the cultural memory of HIV/AIDS from various perspectives. Some edited books adhere to the same line as this but differ in content and frameworks. Indeed, research outputs reveal little interdisciplinary exploration that establishes a dialogue between the revision of HIV/AIDS and the field of cultural memory. Hence, there is substantial scope for research on this nexus, which would establish the base for further development. Academic works on the analysis of cultural representation include *Representations of HIV/AIDS: Visibility Blue/s* by Gabriel Griffin (2001). Griffin suggests that changes in the understanding of HIV/AIDS, the shift from 'dying from the disease' to 'living with it' in Western cultures, and the lack of attention to the impact of HIV/AIDS in several African and Asian countries have caused the 'death' of the disease in the Western media. In *Breaking the Silence: South African Representations of HIV/AIDS* (2013), Ellen Grünkemeier analyses the South African HIV/AIDS pandemic through a number of cultural representations, including novels, photography, films, cartoons, and murals under the framework of literary, cultural, and postcolonial studies. The analysis highlights the role that narratives and visual art have in producing new meanings and influencing the understanding of HIV/AIDS at a social level. The representation of HIV/AIDS through visual arts has been very prolific since the beginning of the pandemic, and this has led to the production of a large number of studies that focus on this discipline. Visual arts have served as a form of individual expression but have also been linked to HIV/AIDS campaigns and collective activism. *Positive Images: Gay Men and HIV/AIDS in the Culture of Post Crisis* by Dion Kagan (2018) examines how the relationship between gay men and HIV has transformed in the past two decades. The author explores literature, film, TV, documentaries, and news coverage from across the English-speaking world to unearth the socio-cultural foundations underpinning this 'post-crisis' period. Mariah Larsson and Elisabet Björklund focus in their edited book on visual arts and use a medical humanities framework to explore the influence of historical representations of HIV/AIDS and stigma in *A Visual History of HIV/AIDS: Exploring the Face of AIDS Film Archive* (2018). *Literary and Visual Representations of HIV/AIDS: Forty Years Later* by Aimee Pozorski, Jennifer J. Lavoie, and Christine J. Cynn (2019) examines representations of the pandemic arguing that literature constitutes a very powerful response to AIDS that ripples into film and politics, driving the changes in past and contemporary representations of HIV/AIDS. Another recent publication, *Disclosures: Rewriting the Narrative about HIV*, edited by Angie Spoto (2018), is an anthologised work from those affected by HIV in Scotland.

Although there has been continuity in the study of HIV/AIDS in critical studies, it is from the first decade of the twenty-first century that we notice an increase in works that include areas of Africa and Latin America, although they are still scarce. While studies on Africa focus on different artistic representations, several studies show that music is central as a form of expression, healing, and resistance for those affected by HIV/AIDS; for example in South Africa, *The Culture of AIDS in Africa: Hope and Healing Through Music and the Arts* (2011) by Gregory Barz and Judah M. Cohen; Uganda, *Singing For Life HIV/AIDS and Music in Uganda* (2014) by Gregory Barz; or Gambia, *Music, Health, and Power: Singing the Unsayable in The Gambia* (2019) by Bonnie B. McConnell. Analysis of cultural representations of Latin America includes *Representations of HIV/AIDS in Contemporary Hispano-American and Caribbean Culture: Cuerpos SuiSIDAs* (2016) and the edited volume *HIV in World Cultures: Three Decades of Representation* (2016), both by Gustavo Subero; and *Viral Voyages Tracing AIDS in Latin America* (2014) by Lina Meruane, who identifies contemporary narratives of 'HIV-Positive Writing' including novels, short stories, urban chronicles, plays, and autobiographical pieces written by mostly gay Latin American authors. In recent years, many journal articles have been published that examine literary works and films, among other narratives, and single-topic special issues have also been published, such as one dedicated to the television series *It's a Sin* (2023) edited by Angelos Bollas.

This edited volume includes contributions from different scholars around the world who focus on the presence and representations of HIV/AIDS in different countries and its peoples, including Cuba, Ireland, South African communities, the United Kingdom, and the United States.

In Chap. 2, Angelos Bollas focuses on the complex portrayal of HIV/AIDS as a form of social suffering in media representations, offering a nuanced examination of how these portrayals shape public perception and policy. Through a detailed analysis of cultural representations, social experiences, and political processes, the chapter critiques the commodification of suffering in the media, highlighting how narratives of those living with

HIV/AIDS are often appropriated to create a spectacle that distances audiences from the authentic experiences of sufferers. Significantly, the chapter draws on the works of Kleinman et al. (1997), as well as other key scholars, to unravel the dynamics of stigmatisation and the construction of social suffering within the socio-cultural context of HIV/AIDS. Bollas argues for a transformation in media representation, advocating for portrayals that emphasise the humanity of sufferers over their affliction, thereby fostering a more inclusive and empathetic understanding. The chapter not only underscores the potential of media to redefine public engagement with social issues but also discusses the critical role of narrative structures and visual strategies in bridging the gap between passive observation and active engagement. This leads to a compelling argument for a media landscape that not only informs but inspires collective responsibility and action towards the alleviation of social suffering. The chapter's exploration of the 'politics of pity' and the implications of media representation in crafting societal norms and moral benchmarks is particularly illuminating. It extends the discourse beyond the realm of academic analysis to real-world implications, emphasising the transformative power of media in shaping societal responses to HIV/AIDS and social suffering at large. This chapter provides a critical lens through which to view the role of media in the societal understanding and response to HIV/AIDS and offers insightful suggestions for more responsible and impactful media practices.

In Chap. 3, Janey Umback critically examines the portrayal of female caregivers in the backdrop of the early HIV/AIDS crisis in Britain, as depicted in Russell T Davies' miniseries, *It's a Sin*. The chapter uniquely focuses on the character of Jill Baxter, inspired by Davies' real-life friend Jill Nalder, an actor and HIV/AIDS activist. Despite the social media trend #BeMoreJill, the chapter highlights the character's underdevelopment, arguing that this mirrors the historical invisibility of female caregivers during the HIV/AIDS crisis. This insightful analysis engages deeply with the portrayal of caregiving in the series, arguing that popular television significantly shapes public perceptions of HIV/AIDS. The narrative of Jill Baxter is used as a lens to explore broader themes of female caregiving, visibility, and the role of media in both reflecting and shaping social memory. The chapter asserts that the series, while successful in bringing to light certain aspects of the LGBTQIA+ experience during the HIV/AIDS crisis, falls short in fully developing its female characters, particularly those in caregiving roles. Umback further discusses how the media's portrayal often relegates women to the background, reducing them to archetypal roles of support. This chapter challenges this normative trend, advocating for a greater acknowledgement and nuanced representation of women, especially those who played pivotal roles during the HIV/AIDS pandemic. By interweaving academic discourse, media analysis, and examples from *It's a Sin*, the chapter illuminates the often-overlooked experiences and contributions of female caregivers. Moreover, it focuses on the complex interplay of media representation, gender norms, and historical memory in constructing narratives of crises like HIV/AIDS. Towards its conclusion, the chapter reflects on the significance of #BeMoreJill as a social media phenomenon, providing a platform for sharing personal narratives of HIV/AIDS caregiving, thereby expanding the discourse beyond the television screen. This chapter makes a significant contribution to the fields of media studies, gender studies, and public health history, offering a critical perspective on the intersections of gender, caregiving, and representation in the context of a major health crisis. It highlights the need for more inclusive and diverse narratives in media representations, which not only depict the reality of different experiences but also shape public understanding and the memory of historical events.

In Chap. 4, Mirta Suquet offers an in-depth exploration of Miguel Angel Fraga's narrative works, set against the backdrop of the Cuban government's response to the HIV/AIDS pandemic during the 1980s and 1990s. Fraga's experiences as a patient in the *Los Cocos* sanatorium provide a unique perspective on the biopolitical strategies employed by the Cuban state during this period, including forced isolation policies that had profound impacts on public health, human rights, and the psychological well-being of those confined. Through a close analysis of Fraga's fictional and non-fictional writings, Suquet highlights the complex interplay between individual experiences of those living with HIV/AIDS and the overarching macro-politics of state control. Drawing on Michel Foucault's concept of the 'incorrigible', the chapter offers an examination of how individuals with HIV/AIDS were categorised within the Cuban sanatorium system and how Fraga's characters subvert this portrayal by embodying a rebellious spirit against authority. The chapter also explores the theme of 'becoming-child' as a form of political resistance, challenging the enforced infantilisation of patients and advocating for a questioning attitude against established norms. Suquet situates Fraga's work within the broader narrative of HIV/AIDS in Latin America, particularly highlighting the impact of institutional censorship and self-censorship in shaping Cuban literature on the subject. It provides a comprehensive look at the psychological traumas resulting from the confinement policy and how these experiences were represented in Fraga's works. Fraga's narratives are presented as a vivid illustration of the struggles, resilience, and creative resistance of patients within the confines of the sanatorium. These stories not only serve as a means of resisting structural and political violence but also stand as a testament to the memory of HIV/AIDS in Cuba. The chapter underscores the importance of acknowledging and seeking reparations for the victims of these policies from the Cuban government. In its conclusion, the chapter asserts the enduring relevance of Fraga's work in contemporary discourse on Cuba and HIV/AIDS, emphasising its role in shaping perspectives, challenging historical narratives, and creating new meanings around the pandemic. Fraga's narratives are seen as crucial in ensuring that the experiences of those who lived through this period remain a significant part of collective memory and continue to impact future generations' understanding of HIV/AIDS in Cuba.

David O'Mullane, in Chap. 5, engages with the complex relationship between the cultural memory of the AIDS pandemic and its influence on contemporary understandings of gay sexual subcultures, particularly focusing on the practice of cruising. The chapter offers an exploration of three post-crisis cultural artefacts: John Walter's *Alien Sex Club* exhibition, Patrick Moore's book *Beyond Shame*, and the collaborative artist book project *Petite Mort*, which collectively examine how memories of the sexual past shape current discourses around promiscuous public sex. In the first section of the chapter, O'Mullane critiques John Walter's 2015 exhibition *Alien Sex Club*, highlighting how Walter portrays cruising as a risky behaviour linked to HIV transmission. The analysis suggests that Walter, influenced by panic and fear from the early years of the AIDS pandemic, presents cruising spaces as dangerous sites of viral transmission, using art to evoke a state of crisis and reinforce moral judgements about promiscuity. The chapter then shifts to Patrick Moore's *Beyond Shame*, a text that counters the sex-negative view of cruising culture. Moore's work seeks to redeem the memory of New York's cruising spaces, portraying them as radical sites of social transformation. However, O'Mullane points out that Moore's approach idealises these spaces, thus creating a nostalgic and perhaps unrealistic vision of cruising as a form of radical political action. The final section discusses *Petite Mort*, a project that offers a nuanced view of public sex, avoiding the extremes of cautionary tales or romanticised narratives. This collaborative work comprises memories of public sex experiences in New York City, illustrating a diverse range of emotions and experiences related to cruising. *Petite Mort* is seen as embracing the complexity and ambivalence of public sex, acknowledging its impact without succumbing to simplistic judgements or idealisations. Throughout the chapter, the concept of hauntology is used to explain how past events and ideas about the AIDS pandemic continue to influence contemporary attitudes and discourses around gay sexual behaviours. This examination reveals that cultural artefacts, whether they are exhibitions, books, or collaborative projects, play a significant role in shaping and sometimes challenging the prevailing narratives about queer sexuality and public sex. The analysis calls for a balanced approach that recognises the complexity of cruising and its role in the queer experience, moving away from binary perspectives that either demonise or romanticise these practices.

In Chap. 6, Elizabeth Mills explores the experiences of HIV-positive women in Khayelitsha, South Africa, interweaving ethnographic research with medical anthropology and human geography theories. The chapter examines the dynamic relationship between memory, space, and embodiment, focusing on women's recollections of their search for healing amid South Africa's political shifts over the last two decades. The structure of the chapter traces women's illness narratives, their embodied experiences of inequality, and their memories in different spatial and temporal contexts. Mills opens the chapter by setting the scene, acknowledging South Africa's significant progress in HIV treatment and the challenges faced during the early 2000s due to government denialism. The research focuses on women activists' role in advocating for HIV treatment in the public health system. The chapter draws parallels with similar anthropological studies, emphasising the unexpected aspects of ethnographic research and the power of imagination in shaping the future of HIV-positive individuals. Mills then focuses on the intersection of race, class, and gender in South Africa and how these dimensions affect health outcomes, even with the large-scale rollout of antiretroviral therapy (ARV). The chapter offers a discussion about the collaborative relationship between the government and activist organisations like the Treatment Action Campaign (TAC), highlighting how socio-economic inequalities impact health. One of the central themes is the fluidity of memory and its construction. The chapter employs the concept of anamnesis, which involves remembrance and the collection of forgotten experiences, to explore how memories shape the present and future. It focuses on women's recollections of embodied precarity linked to HIV and AIDS therapies, using 'precarity' to denote the intersection of socio-economic inequalities with gender, race, class, and age. The methodological approach of the chapter is based on multi-sited ethnography conducted over a long period, with a focus on women in Khayelitsha who played a crucial role in the movement for ARV access. The research methods included interviews, participant photography, and body mapping, among others. Mills examines three 'topologies' of memory, starting with women's narratives of their early lives in the Eastern Cape, and she discusses the socio-spatial construction of gender through rites of passage and the impact of these cultural practices on gender roles and expectations. In the final section, Mills addresses women's memories of navigating different healing practices and health resources in the Eastern and Western Cape provinces to sustain their lives and those of their children. In conclusion, the chapter argues that memories are spatialised and constantly renegotiated through anamnesis, shaping and reshaping people's experiences of illness, health, and life. It emphasises the importance of recognising the unexpected and the power of imagination in understanding and addressing the experiences of HIV-positive individuals. The chapter contributes to the understanding of how place and memory are intertwined in the bodies and narratives of individuals, particularly in the context of HIV/AIDS in South Africa.

In the final chapter (Chap. 7) of this collection, Denise Proudfoot and Ellie Marley discuss the experiences of women and mothers living with HIV (WLHIV and MLHIV), focusing on the gendered implications of an HIV diagnosis and the maternal HIV experience. The chapter draws from qualitative research interviews conducted with Irish-based mothers living with HIV, contextualised within historical, cultural, and sociological frameworks. The chapter highlights that women with HIV come from diverse backgrounds and face unique challenges, particularly in relation to motherhood. The authors first acknowledge the global context of women in the HIV pandemic and the lack of attention given to their specific experiences, especially regarding motherhood. They point out the diverse backgrounds of WLHIV, emphasising that HIV affects women differently than men and that motherhood adds complexity to their experience with HIV. The discussion then moves to the specific issues faced by mothers living with HIV. It critiques the biomedical success in HIV treatment for not addressing the broader implications of the diagnosis, such as emotional and psychological effects and the persistent stigma surrounding HIV. Mothering with HIV is presented as a multifaceted experience, influenced by the availability of highly active antiretroviral therapy (HAART) and societal views on motherhood and HIV. The chapter continues with a discussion of the challenges faced by WLHIV in decision-making around pregnancy and motherhood, including fears of vertical transmission (HIV transmission from mother to child) and societal stigma. Proudfoot and Marley also examine the cultural and societal expectations of women, particularly in Ireland, in relation to motherhood. They discuss how an HIV diagnosis can disrupt the expected life journey towards motherhood, creating a 'biographical disruption'. The experiences of mothers during different eras of the HIV pandemic, from the early years of limited treatment options to the current era of Undetectable = Untransmittable (U=U), are explored. Attention is given to the early years of HIV in Ireland, focusing on the impact on women, especially those in socially deprived areas or involved in drug use. The authors note the significant losses experienced by mothers of children who died from AIDS-related conditions and the lack of societal sympathy due to stigma. The research section presents findings from a study with Irish-based MLHIV. It highlights the diverse backgrounds of the participants and their varied experiences with HIV diagnosis, motherhood, and coping strategies. The study's narrative approach facilitates understanding of the participants' experiences, focusing on their personal, interpersonal, positional, and ideological narratives. Key themes from the research include the shock and unexpected nature of the HIV diagnosis, concerns about vertical transmission, the challenges of disclosure, and the benefits of motherhood in coping with HIV. The authors emphasise the importance of understanding the maternal HIV experience and the need for more women-centred qualitative research focusing on mothering with HIV. In conclusion, Proudfoot and Marley call for increased attention to the unique experiences of women and mothers living with HIV. They underscore the importance of addressing the gendered aspects of the HIV pandemic and advocate for a broader understanding of the challenges faced by WLHIV and MLHIV beyond the medical perspective.

The cultural memory of HIV/AIDS denotes the collective understandings or constructions of the distant past, as people hold them in a given social and historical context. Focusing on cultural representations and the impact on culture vis-à-vis HIV/AIDS, this edited volume explores the significance and the effect of different discourses of the past, the present, and their implications for the future of the HIV pandemic. Narratives on this subject have evolved and led to new debates arising from the reassessment of a pandemic that continues to resonate globally today, albeit differently from its early years.

References

Ajayi, A.I., Abioye, A.O., Adeniyi, O.V., and Akpan, W. 2019. Concerns about contracting HIV, knowing partners' HIV sero-status and discussion of HIV/STI with sexual partners as determinants of uptake of HIV testing. *Journal of Biosocial Science* 51 (4). https://doi.org/10.1017/S0021932018000330.

Adeniyi, Ntombana Rala, and Daniel Ter Goon. 2019. Low Awareness and Use of Pre Exposure Prophylaxis Among Adolescents and Young Adults in High HIV and Sexual Violence Prevalence Settings. *Medicine* 98 (43). https://doi.org/10.1097/MD.0000000000017716.

Barz, Gregory. 2014. *Singing for Life HIV/AIDS and Music in Uganda*. New York: Routledge. https://doi.org/10.4324/9781315024547.

Barz, Gregory, and Judah Cohen. 2011. *The Culture of AIDS in Africa: Hope and Healing Through Music and the Arts*. Oxford: Oxford Academic. https://doi.org/10.1093/acprof:osobl/9780199744473.001.0001.

Bekker, Linda Gail. 2023. The HIV Epidemic 40 years on. *Nature Reviews Microbiology* 21 (12): 767–768. https://doi.org/10.1038/s41579-023-00979-y.

Beyrer, Chris. 2021. A Pandemic Anniversary: 40 Years of HIV/AIDS. *Perspectives, The Art of Medicine* 397 (10290): 2142–2143. https://doi.org/10.1016/S0140-6736(21)01167-3.

Bollas, Angelos. 2023. *It's a Sin* Special Issue. *Journal of Popular Television* 11 (3).

Bond, Lucy, and Jessica Rapson. 2014. *The Transcultural Turn. Interrogating Memory Between and Beyond*. Berlin: Walter de Gruyter.

Brunow, Dagmar. 2015. *Remediating Transcultural Memory: Documentary Filmmaking as Archival Intervention*. Berlin: De Gruyter. https://doi.org/10.1515/9783110436372.

Calabrese, S.K., T.C. Willie, R.W. Galvao, M. Tekeste, J.F. Dovidio, C.B. Safon, O. Blackstock, T. Taggart, C. Kaplan, A. Caldwell, and T.S. Kershaw. 2019. Current US Guidelines for Prescribing HIV Pre-Exposure Prophylaxis (Prep) Disqualify Many Women Who are at Risk and Motivated to Use PrEP. *Journal of Acquired Immune Deficiency Syndromes* 81 (4): 395–405.

CDC. 1981. Kaposi's Sarcoma and Pneumocystis Pneumonia among homosexual men – New York City and California. *MMWR*, 30 (25): 305–308.

Chigwedere, P., G.R. Seage, S. Gruskin, T.H. Lee, and M. Essex. 2008. Estimating the Lost Benefits of Antiretroviral Drug Use in South Africa. *Journal of*

Acquired Immune Deficiency Syndromes 49 (4): 410–415. https://doi.org/10.1097/qai.0b013e31818a6cd5.

Erll, Astrid. 2011. Travelling Memory. *Parallax* 17 (4): 4–18. https://doi.org/10.1080/13534645.2011.605570.

Griffin, Gabriel. 2001. *Representations of HIV/AIDS: Visibility Blue/s.* Manchester: Manchester University Press.

Grimshaw, Ceilidh, Lynsey Boyd, Matt Smith, Claudia S. Estcourt, and Rebecca Metcalfe. 2021. Evaluation of an Inner City HIV Pre-Exposure Prophylaxis Service Tailored to the Needs of People Who Inject Drugs. *HIV Medicine* 22 (10): 965–970.

Grünkemeier, Ellen. 2013. *Breaking the Silence South African Representations of HIV/AIDS.* Woodbridge: James Currey, Boydell and Brewer.

Halbwachs, Maurice. 1992. *On Collective Memory.* Chicago: University of Chicago Press.

He, Na, and Roger Detels. 2005. The HIV Epidemic in China: History, Response, and Challenge. *Cell Res* 15: 825–832. https://doi.org/10.1038/sj.cr.7290354.

HIV/AIDS (UNAIDS). 2022. *Review of UNAIDS Global AIDS Update 2022.* Geneva: Joint United Nations Programme on HIV/AIDS. https://www.unaids.org/en/resources/documents/2022/in-danger-global-aids-update.

———. n.d. Pre-Exposure Prophylaxis Use Expands, but Not Fast Enough. https://www.unaids.org/en/resources/presscentre/featurestories/2022/januay/20220117_preexposure-prophylaxis-use-expands.

Jackson, Kristopher J., Sandra I. McCoy, and Douglas A.E. White. 2023. A Decade of HIV Preexposure Prophylaxis (PrEP): Overcoming Access Barriers in the United States Through Expanded Delivery. *Public Health Reports.* https://doi.org/10.1177/00333549231208487.

Kagan, Dion. 2018. *Positive Images: Gay Men and HIV AIDS in the Culture of Post Crisis.* London: Bloomsbury.

Karris, Maile Y., Susan E. Beekmann, Sanjay R. Mehta, Christy M. Anderson, and Philip M. Polgreen. 2014. Are We Prepped for Preexposure Prophylaxis (PrEP)? Provider Opinions on the Real-World Use of PrEP in the United States and Canada. *Clinical Infectious Diseases* 58 (5): 704–712.

Kleinman, Arthur, Veena Das, and Margaret M. Lock. 1997. Introduction. In *Social Suffering*, ed. Arthur Kleinman, Veena Das, and Margaret M. Lock, ix–xxvii. Berkeley: University of California Press.

Larsson, Mariah, and Elisabet Björklund. 2018. *A Visual History of HIV/AIDS: Exploring the Face of AIDS Film Archive.* London: Routledge.

McConnell, Bonnie B. 2019. *Music, Health, and Power: Singing the Unsayable in the Gambia.* Oxon: Routledge.

Meruane, Lina. 2014. *Viral Voyages Tracing AIDS in Latin America.* New York: Palgrave Macmillan.

Moran, J. 2001. Childhood Sexuality and Education: The Case of Section 28. *Sexualities* 4 (1): 73–89.

Nagourney, Adam. 2023. *The Times*. New York: Crown Publishing Group.

Nora, Piere. 1989. Between Memory and History: Les Lieux de Mémoire. *Representations* 26: 7–24.

Pintado Gutiérrez, Lucía, and Alicia Castillo Villanueva. 2019. *New Approaches to Translation, Conflict, and Memory: Narratives of the Spanish Civil War and the Dictatorship*. Cham: Palgrave Macmillan. https://doi.org/10.1007/978-3-030-00698-3.

Pozorski, Aimee, Jennifer J. Lavoie, and Christine J. Cynn. 2019. *Literary and Visual Representations of HIV/AIDS: Forty Years Later*. London: Lexington Book, Rowman & Littlefield.

Robinson, Shirleene. 2014. Beyond Tombstones and Grim Reapers: The Gay Community's Challenge to Official HIV/AIDS Campaigns in 1980s Australia and Britain. In *Acts of Love and Lust*, ed. Lisa Featherstone, Rebecca Jennings, and Robert Reynolds, 95–111. Newcastle upon Tyne: Cambridge Scholars Publishing.

Shilts, Randy. 2011. *And the Band Played on: Politics, People, and the AIDS Epidemic*. Chicago: Souvenir Press.

Simelela, Nono, W.D. Francois Venter, Yogan Pillay, and Peter Barron. 2015. A Political and Social History of HIV in South Africa. *Current HIV/AIDS Reports* 12 (2): 256–261. https://doi.org/10.1007/s11904-015-0259-7.

Spieldenner, Andrew. 2016. PrEP Whores and HIV Prevention: The Queer Communication of HIV Pre-Exposure Prophylaxis (PrEP). *Journal of Homosexuality* 63 (12): 1685–1697.

Spoto, Angie. 2018. *Disclosures: Rewriting the Narrative about HIV*. Edinburgh: Stewed Rhubarb Press.

Stacey, Jackie. 1991. Promoting Normality: Section 28 and the Regulation of Sexuality. In *Off-Centre: Feminism and Cultural Studies*, ed. Sarah Franklin, Celia Lury, and Jackie Stacey, 284–320. London: HarperCollins.

Subero, Gustavo. 2016a. *HIV in World Cultures: Three Decades of Representation*. Farnham: Ashgate.

———. 2016b. *Representations of HIV/AIDS in Contemporary Hispano-American and Caribbean Culture: Cuerpos SuiSIDAs*. Farnham: Ashgate.

Thomson, Rachel. 1993. Unholy Alliances: The Recent Politics of Sex Education. In *Activating Theory: Lesbian, Gay, Bisexual Politics*, ed. Joseph Bristow and Anglia R. Wilson, 219–245. London: Lawrence and Wishart.

UNAIDS. 2023. *The Path that Ends AIDS: UNAIDS Global AIDS Update 2023*. Geneva: Joint United Nations Programme on HIV/AID.

CHAPTER 2

Beyond the Spectacle: Rethinking Media Representations of HIV/AIDS and Social Suffering

Angelos Bollas

2.1 Introduction

In *Social Suffering* (1997), Kleinman, Das, and Lock argue that three themes transpire from representations of social suffering. These are "[...] cultural representations, social experiences, political and professional processes" (xi). Cultural representations of suffering are very common in popular culture as well as in specific social institutions. Such representations make use of visual and aural modalities and include, among others, images—still and/or moving—stories, that almost become archetypal, and linguistic devices as metaphors in everyday life. Cultural representations often establish certain moralities, which, in turn, are used to justify conservative policies and politics. This chapter provides social suffering as a frame through which media representations of HIV/AIDS can be

A. Bollas (✉)
Department of Sociology, Maynooth University, Maynooth, Ireland
e-mail: angelos.bollas@mu.ie

A. Castillo Villanueva, A. Bollas (eds.), *HIV/AIDS in Memory, Culture and Society*, Palgrave Studies in Science and Popular Culture, https://doi.org/10.1007/978-3-031-59699-5_2

analysed with attention to how social suffering, as a trope, is used as a tool which aids social regulation. To illustrate this, one need only consider the function of the HIV/AIDS retrovision genre, a media product offering a perspective that intertwines various emotions towards the past, oscillating between a sense of dismay when recalling instances of brutality and suppression, and a wistful longing for a bygone era marked by innocence and elegance (Kagan 2018, 166–167). Recycling an anachronistic perception of the reality of the HIV-positive person and the society within which this person lives can often nurture conservative ideologies. Audiences of such representations can be encouraged to ignore contemporary advances in science and succumb to the fear and social prejudice of the past.[1] Therefore, by means of cultural representations, social suffering becomes part of social experience. If, in other words, we accept that experience is not inherited but learned, then cultural representations can be considered to be a way through which experience is learned, norms are created, and thereupon normalised. Ultimately, changing how HIV/AIDS and broader social suffering are portrayed in media involves reshaping how stories and images are presented. Focusing on the human aspect of sufferers rather than just their conditions can lead to greater empathy and inclusivity. Additionally, reducing the distance between viewer and subject in media can turn passive viewership into active participation, encouraging a media environment that prompts collective action and responsibility in addressing social suffering.

Societal and cultural changes impact our understanding of fundamental aspects of human identity and experience. Kleinman et al. (1997, xii) argue that "[e]ven what we so easily assume to be the existential ground of the human condition [...] may undergo change in keeping with epochal transformations in the nexus of symbolic-moral systems and the political economy [...]". Here, the authors further illustrate how even what is considered to be the core of human existence is not as significant as it might be thought to be. A case in point is the constitution of masculinity, which is erroneously thought to be a universal invariable but, in fact, is dynamic and oscillates in accordance with its socio-cultural context (Bollas 2021). Based on the relationship between cultural representations and social

[1] Kleinman et al. (1997, p. xi) further argue that the establishment of such historical memories of suffering also contributes to the commodification of suffering. Even though this is evident in our current society and the way PrEP is being marketed, this is not the focus of this section and, therefore, I will not expand on this further.

experience that has been discussed so far, one concludes that social suffering is exploited in such a way as to fashion responses to it according to the political and socio-cultural context of a given place and time. Such manipulation of social suffering, Kleinman et al. (1997, xii) argue, involves "[...] political and professional processes [that are] both authorised and contested [...]. Even in seeking to manage social suffering, [these processes] have, through intended and unintended effects, intensified human misery." The workings of homonormative politics attest to this argument. Non-heterosexual individuals populate popular media, purportedly to reduce social discrimination against non-heterosexuals, but the way they are represented results in further stigmatisation of non-heterosexuals who do not conform to heteronormative values (Bollas 2021).

If, therefore, cultural representations define what is—perceived to be—real and what is not, then Kleinman et al. (1997, xii) are right in arguing that "[s]ocial suffering is a feature of cultural representation both as a spectacle and as the presentation of the real." We know of social suffering because it is shown to us; further, we know how to respond to social suffering because this is also shown to us. Reality is mediated through cultural representations, and, as it has already been discussed, what is mediated as real depends on power.[2] The banality of the description of our culture as a visual one comes into play when one considers that the way we visually represent social suffering becomes the way social suffering is imagined to be. "The very act of picturing distorts social experience in the popular media and in the professions under the impress of ideology and political economy" (xiii). Reality is transformed both for the spectators of social suffering and for the sufferers themselves. Kleinman et al. (1997, xiii) ask,

> Is that transformation anamorphic in the sense of a greater experience of complexity, or is it anamorphic in the sense that the global lenses of the media and other transnational institutions distort local images while providing the optical system for regularising (normalising) the global recovery of images and experiences?

In cultural representations of HIV/AIDS, the latter seems to prevail. From *Philadelphia* (1993) to *The Next Best Thing* (2000) to *The Line of*

[2] Mitchell (1994) writes about the ethics of representation and focuses on the relationship between representation and responsibility, arguing that this relationship constitutes a major moral dilemma of contemporary life.

Beauty (2006) to *Dallas Buyers Club* (2013), representations of HIV/AIDS have been contributing to the creation of a cultural memory of HIV/AIDS which normalises types of social suffering as well as responses to it.[3] Who is to be pitied, who is to receive help, and who is to be deemed deserving of their suffering is dictated by the ways in which social suffering is depicted in these representations.[4] If the language of representation dictates—and/or distorts—reality, then it must be through this very language of representation that change can occur.[5] In other words, to prevent distortioned understandings of social suffering, one has to modify the way language is used in cultural representations of social suffering to define, illustrate, and present it more accurately. By appropriating practices of mediation and offering a greater plurality of representations of people living with HIV/AIDS (PLWHA), it is more likely that an accurate picture of the reality of life with HIV/AIDS can be painted. Indeed, "[...] cultural representations of suffering [...] authorise transformations of core symbol systems and cultural discourses and thereby alter social experience, inducing ominous historical change in experiences of suffering in our own epoch" (Kleinman et al. 1997, xviii). As such, ideal representations would be those which destabilise the trivialisation of suffering, reverse the romanticised version of the victim as a hero, and expose the workings of power in the construction, mediated or otherwise, of social suffering.[6]

2.2 Suffering and Representation

Kleinman and Kleinman (1997) argue that "[the] existential appeal of human experiences, their potential to mobilise popular sentiment and collective action, and even their capability to witness or offer testimony are

[3] For an in-depth analysis of these productions, see Kagan (2018).

[4] In line with the Denver Principles, it is important to note that the use of the words suffering and sufferers in this chapter refers only to cultural productions that present HIV/AIDS and PLWHA within discourses and contexts of suffering.

[5] I use the word language to refer to the means through which representation is realised, that is, images, body language, gestures, words, looks, subtext, etc.

[6] This 'trivialisation of suffering' in cultural products is achieved in a number of ways. There have been works focusing on HIV/AIDS the publicity of which did not mention HIV/AIDS at all (e.g., Aron's *The Stanley Parkers* (1990)). Also, in theatre, for a very long time, there had been plays insisting on not portraying AIDS-caused deaths on stage; or plays in which only offstage characters died with AIDS (e.g., Deegan's *The Queen and Peacock* (2000)). For more information about HIV/AIDS in theatre, see Singleton (2011) and O'Brian (2017).

now available for gaining market share" (1). Observing the circulation of the visual representation of suffering among both local and global audiences/markets, Kleinman and Kleinman's argument here highlights the commercialisation of suffering, which presupposes the commodification of experience. It should be noted that commercialising experiences of suffering can have positive outcomes as long as it occurs in a manner that is not exploitative or stigmatising. Bollas (2022, 2023) offers examples of positive representations of HIV/AIDS as social suffering in works such as *Pose* (2018–2021) and *It's a Sin* (2021), where 'suffering' is not operationalised to spread fear and panic but is used in a manner that accentuates the societal mistreatment of PLWHA. However, when representations of suffering are distortive, by which I mean when they use the trope of social suffering to further stigmatise PLWHA and not to address issues of systemic discrimination, the experience of suffering becomes a commodity. As with all media representations, audience/markets are not presented with the reality of this experience per se; rather, they are presented with a version of said reality. Reality is, thus, re-told, re-enacted, re-performed, and the experience of suffering becomes replicated. What the audience is presented with is not the experience of suffering but an imitation of that experience. It is during the process of creating the representation, the imitation of reality, where an experience of suffering is turned into a commodity and, therefore, can be manipulated in any way that can maximise its commodity value. Kleinman and Kleinman (1997) further observe that suffering "[…] is routinely appropriated in American popular culture, which is a leading edge of global popular culture" (2). The representation of a staged, thus possibly distorted, version of social suffering reminds us of the Platonic ***simulacrum***. For Plato, representations of reality had to be distorted so that they could be considered to be as real(istic) as possible.

To illustrate his point, Plato used statuary as an example. To ensure an accurate representation for the viewer, the top part of a sculpture had to be larger than the bottom one. To the viewer, this created the illusion that the statue was an accurate representation of real life. Had the same sculpture been viewed in scale, its deformity would have been obvious. With this metaphor, Plato highlighted the fact that a distortion can be perceived as truth if representation of an object is manipulated in such a way as to create a real(istic) effect. In modernity, Baudrillard (1994) extends Plato's view on representation and suggests the following four types, viewed either as individual phases or a continuum: a faithful imitation of reality; a representation of reality, based on reality, that aims to conceal its flaws; a representation of reality which is not based on reality but pretends to be the reality itself; and a presentation of reality which is based on a representation of what ought to be real and is so far removed from reality that is not related to reality at all. The last is what Baudrillard defines as *simulacrum*.[7]

What is achieved by a *simulacrum* of social suffering? What end is served through the manipulation of experience for the sake of representation? And how does the cultural appropriation of social suffering through representation contribute to the prescription of socio-cultural responses to social suffering? Sontag (2003), though focusing on war photography, questions the effectiveness of suffering-related images in eliciting a genuine reaction of compassion from viewers, by discussing how repeated exposure to images of suffering can lead to desensitisation. The more one is exposed to a mediated form of suffering, the more indifferent one might become to the actual suffering that is represented. She also raises questions about the voyeuristic aspect of looking at photos of people in pain and the potential for such images to exploit their subjects. Kleinman and Kleinman (1997) describe a process whereby sufferers, through the narrativisation of their suffering, are reduced to their trauma stories, further reduced into victims, and from this corralling into victimisation, they become patients. More specifically, Kleinman and Kleinman (1997, 9–10, emphasis in original) write about sufferers for whom "[...] their intimately interior images of violation are made over into *trauma stories.* [...] Increasingly, those complicated stories, based on real events, [are] reduced to a core cultural image of *victimisation* [...]. Then, [the victim] becomes a patient [...]." The pathologisation of suffering, as described by this quote, might indeed be a way for sufferers to claim financial and other benefits. It could, therefore, be a transformation they actively seek out in order to survive.

Following the development and fights of early AIDS activism in the States, for example, allows us to understand how representation of suffering became an objective of activists since this was an effective way for sufferers to be provided with medical, moral, and possibly financial support. However, a closer examination of early societal and political responses to HIV/AIDS provides a clearer understanding of how the representation of

[7] I draw on Baudrillard's work to highlight the levels and layers of distortion reality go through in the process of representation. For an in-depth discussion on Baudrillard's work, see Redhead's (2008) excellent study on Baudrillard.

HIV/AIDS as social suffering created a *simulacrum* whereby the identity of the sufferer was distorted. Rather than perceiving the HIV positive or the AIDS patient as the person who suffers, representations of suffering created a discourse very different to the reality of suffering. AIDS patients, along with those who were potential AIDS patients, were viewed as a threat to social order, to health, and to morality. The sufferers were not the HIV-positive people or the AIDS patients anymore, but those who were not infected but had the potential to be. Representation created a *simulacrum* within which stigmatisation flourished on grounds that were completely justified in the consciousness of the many.

Examples of this can be found in the discourses of moral panic that started with the outbreak of the epidemic, whereby HIV-positive individuals were described as the "[...] AIDS carriers [...]," those who can potentially infect the rest of the population (Altman 2001, 145). In such narratives, the sufferer was not the HIV positive or AIDS-infected individual; rather, the sufferer was the one who was in danger of being infected by the amoral AIDS carrier. Those who were not infected were creating narratives of victimhood.[8] So, on the one hand, using cultural appropriations to situate HIV/AIDS social suffering within medical terms allowed HIV positive and AIDS patients access to medical and moral/social care and support. On the other hand, as Simon Watney (1987, 3, emphasis in original) explains, representations of HIV/AIDS resulted in HIV/AIDS "[...] being used as a pretext throughout the West to 'justify' calls for increasing legislation and regulation of those who are considered to be socially unacceptable." In the HIV/AIDS suffering *simulacrum*, the roles of the one who suffers the impact of HIV/AIDS and the one who does not are reversed.

The appropriation of social suffering does not occur only through the construction and circulation of a language of representation via channels of cultural consumption. Such an appropriation, and quite possibly one of more overt political significance, can also be achieved through the absence of representation. "The absent image is also a form of political appropriation," Kleinman and Kleinman (1997, 17) note; "public silence is perhaps more terrifying than being overwhelmed by public images of atrocity." In the history of HIV/AIDS, there have been two periods in which this public silence was especially evident: the first was at the outbreak of the epidemic, and the second from the late 1990s to the early 2010s. Both

[8] For a detailed discussion on how AIDS was initially narrativised, see Patton (1990).

instances of public silence attempted to render HIV/AIDS as well as PLWHA non-existent. Patton (1990, 3), discussing the early years of the epidemic, describes silencing as the "[...] discursive effect symptomatic of relations of power," suggesting what has already been argued here and in the previous chapter: the silencing of HIV/AIDS as social suffering was not a sign of ignorance but a sign of conscious and strategic attempt to erase, metaphorically and potentially literally, the experience of the particular suffering and the sufferers themselves. In *Inventing AIDS* (1990), Patton describes the early years of the epidemic as a constant battle for representation. On the one hand, media and governments pretended to be ignorant about an epidemic which was killing an exponentially growing number of people; on the other hand, activists were trying to bring the public's attention to HIV/AIDS as social suffering. The aim was "[...] to promote compassion and decrease irrational fear [...]" (9). The years that followed saw an increased interest in broadcasting anything HIV/AIDS-related to the point that media representations gave rise to social and moral panics related to HIV and AIDS.[9]

The second instance of silence, which lasted significantly longer than the first one, followed the invention of combination therapy and highly active antiretroviral therapies (HAART). Kagan (2018) observes that from 1996 until the mid-2010s, cultural representations of HIV/AIDS were few and far between. It can be argued that the reasons for the second erasure of HIV/AIDS from cultural representations served, yet again, homonormative political agendas. Similar to the initial cultural erasure of HIV/AIDS, which aided the inscription of HIV/AIDS as a social rather than a medical problem, the second attempt to erase it served the neoliberal homonormative agenda, whereby the fight for marriage equality could not be undermined by images which linked homosexuality to deviance. With the pretext of HIV/AIDS being treatable, attention on HIV/AIDS diminished in, at least, the Western Anglophone popular culture. Both instances of silencing, the one caused by conservative governments and the one stemming from conservative political agendas of neoliberal gay activists, were equally dangerous. Kleinman and Kleinman (1997, 17) note that the "[...] official silence is another form of appropriation [...] it prevents public witnessing." They further add that when such erasures occur, "[...] the possibility of moral appeal through images of human

[9] Both Patton (1990) and Watney (1987) offer a critical analysis of the political and socio-cultural responses to HIV and AIDS.

misery is prevented, and it is their absence that is the source of existential dismay" (16). In other words, not only is the possibility of distorting the experience of suffering in the public arena looming over the silencing of suffering but, most importantly, such an erasure of experience results in the intensification of suffering itself.

2.3 Instances of Representation and Silencing of Social Suffering

When analysing instances of cultural appropriation of suffering, we must spread our attention equally to instances of representation as well as instances of absence of representation. Kleinman and Kleinman (1997) wonder about the significance of representations, or the lack of representations, of social suffering.

> To what uses are experiences of suffering put? What are the consequences of those cultural practices for understanding and responding to human problems? And what are the more general implications of the cultural appropriations of suffering for human experience, including human experiences of suffering? (3).

To address these questions, we must first visualise how the observation and/or experience of—mediated—social suffering occurs. The very staging of the experience of social suffering requires two parties: the sufferers and those who are present in the scenes of suffering but do not directly experience suffering themselves. Further to these two parties present at the scene of suffering are those who aid the mediation process. For example, when considering the staging of HIV/AIDS in the TV adaptation of *Angels in America* (2003), we should not only think of the characters who are present in the scene of suffering. We should also consider producers, production managers, production assistants, HBO, companies who advertise their products while the series airs, and others who are not only involved in but also benefit financially and otherwise from the representation of suffering.

Therefore, representations of suffering can become exploitative insofar as those who do not suffer gain from it, while the ones who actually experience suffering neither gain from nor participate in the process of representation. Despite the fact that the creative team might include PLWHA, the people whose story is staged are almost never the ones who profit from the telling of their story. They are stripped of any role in narrating because it is not they who share their stories of suffering but actors, writers, directors, editors, and other creatives. This has been one of the major criticisms of works such as *Paris is Burning* (1990), which documented the suffering of PLWHA. The creators of the documentary gave a nominal fee instead of what they would consider to be a fair share of the profits to those whose suffering became the focus of the documentary (Green 1993). Kleinman and Kleinman (1997, 8) confirm that "[we] gain in moral status and some of our organisations gain financially and politically, while those whom we represent, or appropriate, remain where they are, moribund, surrounded by vultures."

To aid the development of my argument, I summon Bourdieu's theory of social fields to argue that the act of representation of social suffering creates a social field in which the one who suffers and the one who does not are positioned in a relationship of power (Hilgers and Mangez 2014). The former (the sufferer) is rendered at best powerless and at worst silenced, while the one who does not experience the suffering, but benefits from it, is rendered powerful. Here, it is important to note that this social field does not include the audience; rather, it aims to describe the scene of suffering as a *locus* where unequal power relations are formed. Both the sufferer and the one who is present at the scene of suffering, but does not actually suffer, refer to the agents who make up the scene of suffering in cultural productions.

To further my argument, I use the term real life in contrast to the *simulacrum* that I discussed earlier. In *real life*, the non-sufferer has power over the one who suffers. In the *simulacrum*, the mediation of reality has reversed the roles of sufferer and non-sufferer. There, the HIV-negative person is presented as the one who is in danger of moral, social, or physical infection by the immoral, irresponsible, and aberrant Other; that is, the HIV-positive one or the one who can potentially become HIV positive. This results in providing the one who has power in real life to use their position of weakness created in the *simulacrum* as an alibi for exercising power over the Other, the one who actually experiences suffering. Within HIV/AIDS history, we have observed such exertions of power in the shape of physical, emotional, and moral violence, as well as social discrimination, stigma, and isolation.

2.4 Identifying with/the Other

The discussions about the sufferer—or the non-sufferer as per the discussion above—so far in the chapter do not refer to a universal sufferer. What people perceive as suffering and, by extension, who they identify as a sufferer largely depends on whether or not they can establish some sort of connection or identification with either the situation of suffering or the sufferer. Morris (1997, 41) observes that suffering "[...] is not a raw datum, a natural phenomenon we can identify and measure, but a social status that we extend or withhold. We extend or withhold it depending largely on whether the sufferer falls within our moral community." Morris focuses on suffering as a social status that is bestowed upon those whose suffering is identified by those who are not experiencing suffering and, thus, have the power to extend or withhold social statuses ad libitum. Morris (1997, 41) further states that we "[...] do not acknowledge the destruction of beings outside our moral community as suffering." This offers an additional justification for my previous argument about the erasure of suffering through the avoidance of representations of it. It emerges that the absence of representation of social suffering signifies an acknowledgement of the sufferer as the Other.

Within the HIV/AIDS history, Kerr (2016), much like Kagan (2018), also observes two periods of such othering through lack of representation. The first one, he argues, refers to the initial 5 years of the epidemic when Ronald Reagan, then President of the United States, refused to utter the word AIDS in public. The second silencing refers to the period starting from 1996 until the end of the first decade of the twenty-first century. Based on Morris's (1997) observations about suffering being a status that mainstream culture assigns or withholds, it is not surprising that the big hit which broke the period of second silencing was the Academy Award-winning and international success *Dallas Buyers Club* (2013), the main character of which was white and heterosexual. Needless to say, this has not been the first or the last time the PLWHA is depicted in a manner that provides opportunities for members of the audience to identify with. *Philadelphia* (1993), arguably the first mainstream film to focus on HIV/AIDS, also presented us with a main character who 'ticks the boxes' of mainstream culture. Andrew Beckett, the main character of the film, is a highly successful lawyer who keeps his homosexuality conveniently in the closet. How could the audience not identify him as a sufferer when he appeared to share so many common characteristics with them? It could be argued that the film's repeated references to the discrimination he faced as a gay man and a person living with HIV/AIDS would make audience identification difficult. However, Beckett illustrates the homonormative ideal of a man who has a respectful job, and even though he is a homosexual, he is not an 'in your face' kind of homosexual, which contributes to making him a more likeable character for the movie's contemporary audience.

The question we need to ask, though, is whether it was the sharing of common characteristics that aided audience identification with him or a hegemonic aspirational dynamic? He was white, upper-class, well-educated, and financially independent. With characteristics like these, he was identified as part of the broader moral community of the time and was extended sufferer status. Morris (1997, 41) observes that representation has the "[...] power to reinvent suffering. [... By] extending or contracting the borders of a moral community, [representation] can be used with different degrees of blindness or insight." Taking the representation of the character of Andrew Beckett as an example, it becomes clear that the borders of the moral community of the spectators were expanded. Because he is represented as white, upper-class, well-educated, and financially independent, he was not perceived as Other but as one of 'us'.[10] Therefore, the borders of the moral community of the spectators were expanded to accept him as a sufferer because, his suffering aside, he embodies mainstream society. Here, it should be highlighted that the diversity of the audience and their ability to read and respond to texts in a variety of ways are not ignored. The discussion about a moral community and mainstream society reflects an acknowledgement of the existence of a dominant, hegemonic worldview that is white, male, and middle class. Therefore, even if one does not belong to what is commonly considered to be mainstream society by being white, male, and middle class, it is very likely, though not absolutely inevitable, that one might have adopted the worldview of mainstream society and, thus, formed a common moral community.

[10] Here, 'us' is used as an aspirational rather than a real category for most audience members.

2.5 Effects of the Mediation of Social Suffering

So far, it has been established that the way we understand and interact with social suffering is very much related to the ways in which suffering is represented or to the significance associated with the absence of representation of suffering in culture. Additionally, the discussion has shown that representations of suffering create power relations and that a thorough understanding of social suffering as a spectacle is very important in examining ways that representation can be used to eliminate social inequalities related to social suffering. As such, the chapter now turns its focus on the socio-cultural and political effects of the mediation of social suffering. If we accept Hannertz's (1996) definition of cosmopolitanism as "[...] an orientation, a willingness to relate with the Other" (103, emphasis in original), we should examine the role of the media in representing the suffering Other and, more importantly, the role of the media in nurturing cosmopolitans. In Chouliaraki's (2006, 2) words, we should examine "[...] the conditions under which it is possible for the media to cultivate an ideal identity for the spectator as a citizen of the world." The very act of mediation is an act of distancing, both physical and otherwise. The previous discussion attests to that distancing: through representation, social suffering becomes a distant state that might concern people with whom we can identify, but it does not affect our immediate environment.

The previous section addressed the representation of social suffering as aiding the accumulation of power for mainstream society. Through the hegemonic Othering of the sufferer, the one who does not experience suffering becomes more powerful and is made to believe that they can exert their power over the ones who suffer. This realisation, though, is not a productive one. It does not offer any insights as to whether representation can be used to subvert established positions of power. It is, therefore, imperative to examine "[...] whether or not the media can cultivate a disposition of care for and engagement with the far away other; whether or not television can create a global public with a sense of social responsibility towards the distant sufferer" (Chouliaraki 2006, 1). If the media can, indeed, be used to raise public awareness of the conditions and implications of social suffering, which, in turn, can lead to the improvement of life for all, then representation can be put to good use.

The starting point of the study of mediation is the examination of the possibilities that each mediation allows with regard to the spectators' reactions to portrayals of suffering. Indeed, one should not assume a homogeneous group when referring to spectators of cultural products. Therefore, rather than speculating how an assumed audience would react to representations of suffering, this study focuses on understanding the array of possible reactions that are elicited from the way a cultural product mediates suffering. A question that is of importance when studying representations of suffering is under what conditions one might feel an urge to act when presented with images of suffering. Chouliaraki (2006) argues that in order for the spectator to develop some sort of sympathy for, and possibly help, the one who experiences suffering, it is vital that both the suffering and its implications be presented to the spectator. In other words, through representations of suffering that are not *simulacra* but are as close to lived experiences as possible, spectators can develop feelings that could motivate them to take action.

Here, it should be noted that action is understood in this project in line with Alexander's (1987, 300) definition as "[...] interpretation and strategization." The former refers to a dialogic relationship between individuals who take for granted that their understanding of the world is the only understanding possible and the change that occurs to that understanding every time individuals encounter understandings that are different to theirs. The latter, strategization, refers to action as more than just understanding the world; it refers to action as "[...] transforming and acting upon it" (302). Surely, strategization appears to be the most significant component of action in that it can more decisively contribute to change. However, I am of the position that interpretation is an equally significant component of action with regard to social suffering in that it is the prerequisite for strategization to occur. What is more, it might not be a realistic expectation of representations of suffering that they elicit action in the form of strategization. Yet, the possibility appears to lie more in creating representations of social suffering that have the capacity to encourage action in the form of interpretation.

There are many questions that loom out of this remark: "[...] under which conditions is it at all possible for the media to induce displays of global care for people we know nothing about and will never meet?" (Chouliaraki 2006, 1). What does it take for a representation of suffering to not just create feelings of pity in spectators but to make them take action, be it reconsidering their own prejudice against PLWHA or actively helping and supporting them? "Do political protest and social solidarity have a place in television's mediations of distant suffering?" (*ibid.*). Also crucial to consider is the very distance between spectator and spectacle that the mediation of suffering creates. Mass media provide spectators with vivid images of suffering upon which, even if the spectators wished to act, the very distance created by the media of representation renders any attempt for action worthless. Chouliaraki confirms that "[...] mass media have intensified the tensions involved in the enactment of public action because they constantly confront us with realities that occur too far away from everyday life for us to feel that we can make a difference to them" (2).[11] The tension that is created between the need of spectators to take action and the inability to do so because of the distance that mediation creates is such that, if intensified, there is the danger that spectators might switch off. In other words, this tension is a significant point for consideration that informs decisions relevant to representation. How suffering is represented, therefore, is affected by that tension. Mediation of suffering must ensure that the tension remains within acceptable limits.

When discussing the strategies involved in moderating the tension that the distance of mediation creates for spectators, Boltanski (1999) explains that representation is constrained so that it can be digested easily by the spectator; this is what Boltanski calls "politics of pity" (7). In unpacking the politics of pity, which will in turn provide a thorough understanding of the staging and mediation of suffering, Chouliaraki (2006) suggests we examine "[...] how the sufferer is portrayed on screen and how the screen of suffering is narrated" (3). This, she continues, can give us access to understand what it is that orientates "[...] the spectator's attitude towards the distant sufferer and, in the long run, [shapes] the disposition of television publics vis-à-vis the misfortune of faraway others" (*ibid.*, emphasis in original).[12] In the previous section, for example, I examined one function of the mediation of suffering: helping communities define themselves as non-sufferers. By watching the suffering of Others, spectators identify themselves as non-sufferers. At the collective level, this might mean that through the suffering of Others, communities of non-sufferers develop a sense of togetherness; a togetherness that is free of suffering because they are in a safe distance from the sufferers. Therefore, "[...] aesthetic narratives of mediation have more to say about the life of spectators than the

[11] Chouliaraki here echoes the work of Ellis (2000) who focused on the moral demands made on spectators by television when presented with images of suffering without being offered the opportunity to do something about it, to act on it.

[12] If we are to truly understand mediation, Silverstone (2004) advises focusing on both the institutions and the technologies through which mediation occurs.

ethical dilemmas that the life of the distant sufferers may press on our societies" (5). Through the representation of social suffering, the role of television becomes one of producing socio-cultural identities. Television, Chouliaraki argues, "[...] construes the nation as an 'imagined' community by homogenising differences internal to the nation state and, similarly, [...] transnational news flows construe a 'beyond the nation' community by establishing of a broader 'we'" (10, emphasis in original).

Focusing on HIV/AIDS, representations of HIV/AIDS contributed to the emergence of a global North sentiment of communal identity among spectators of suffering: despite the possible physical proximity between HIV positive, or potentially positive, and HIV-negative individuals, the cultural landscape in the global North was divided between sufferers and spectators. Spectators who were not part of the sufferers' group grew stronger as a result of that sense of togetherness as a group who do not suffer that is described above. Not only did they have power because they were not part of the sufferers' group, but their power grew because they formed part of a bigger group of those who do not suffer but consume media products that mediate the suffering of Others to satisfy their own emotional gratifications.

2.6 Conclusion

This chapter illustrates the pivotal role cultural representations play in shaping our understanding of social suffering, especially in the context of HIV/AIDS. It emphasises how social suffering as a media frame, through selective emphasis and omission, has historically influenced public perception, crafting a narrative that often distorts the reality of those living with HIV/AIDS. These portrayals have significant implications, including the legitimisation of certain responses to suffering, the perpetuation of stigmatisation, and the formation of policies. As we consider the broader impact of these cultural representations, it becomes apparent that they not only mirror society's prevailing ideologies but also actively contribute to the construction of social reality. The portrayal of HIV/AIDS as social suffering in media, from early cinema to contemporary television, has often oscillated between evoking sympathy and reinforcing stigma, depending on the alignment of the sufferer's image with societal norms and moral benchmarks. This chapter has shown that the *sufferer* is not a static entity but is defined through a dynamic interplay of visibility, representation, and the politics of identification. The silences and vocalisations of suffering in media narratives, as described, are not mere oversights or emphases but are strategic choices that have profound effects on the sufferers and the audience. They shape the moral economy of suffering, dictating who is worthy of empathy and assistance and who is not. The politics of pity, as elucidated, crafts a specific kind of spectatorship—one that may foster a sense of detachment or a superficial engagement with the sufferer's plight rather than a deep moral or ethical commitment to alleviate their suffering.

In closing, it is essential to recognise that the potential for changing the discourse around HIV/AIDS and social suffering at large lies in altering the narrative structures and visual strategies employed in media representations. By challenging the normalised scripts of suffering and engaging with the sufferers' narratives in a manner that foregrounds their humanity over their affliction, we can foster a more inclusive and empathetic understanding. Moreover, by bridging the gap that mediation creates between the sufferer and the spectator, we can transform passive observation into active engagement, paving the way for a media landscape that not only informs but also inspires collective responsibility and action towards the alleviation of social suffering.

References

Alexander, Jeffrey C. 1987. Action and Its Environments. In *The Micro-Macro Link*, ed. Jeffrey C. Alexander, Bernhard Giesen, Richard Münch, and Neil J. Smelser, 288–318. Berkeley: University of California Press.

Altman, Dennis. 2001. *Global Sex.* Chicago: The University of Chicago Press.

Baudrillard, Jean. 1994. *Simulacra and Simulation*, Trans. S. F. Glacer. Ann Arbor: University of Michigan Press.

Bollas, Angelos. 2021. Masculinities on the Side: An Exploration of the Function of Homosexism in Maintaining Hegemonic Masculinities and Sexualities. *Sexuality & Culture* 25: 1761–1770.

———. 2022. Viral Representations in Pose (2018-2021). *Journal of Popular Film and Television* 50 (3): 112–129.

———. 2023. Viral Representations in It's a Sin (2021). *Journal of Popular Television* 11 (2): 135–153.

Boltanski, Luc. 1999. *Distant Suffering: Politics, Morality, and the Media.* Cambridge: Cambridge University Press.

Chouliaraki, Lilie. 2006. *The Spectatorship of Suffering.* London: Sage.

Ellis, John. 2000. *Seeing Things: Television in the Age of Uncertainty.* London: I. B. Tauris.

Green, Jesse. 1993. Paris Has Burned. *The New York Times*, April 18. Available at: https://bit.ly/3CNutbj. Accessed 16 Dec 2020.

Hannertz, Ulf. 1996. *Transnational Connections: Culture, People, Places.* London: Routledge.

Hilgers, Mathieu, and Eric Mangez. 2014. Introduction to Pierre Bourdieu's Theory of Social Fields. In *Bourdieu's Theory of Social Fields: Concepts and Applications*, ed. Mathieu Hilgers and Eric Mangez, 1–36. London: Routledge.

Kagan, Dion. 2018. *Positive Images: Gay Men and HIV/AIDS in The Culture of 'Post-crisis'.* London: I. B. Tauris.

Kerr, Theodore. 2016. AIDS 1969: HIV, History, and Race. *Drain* 13(2). Available at: http://drainmag.com/aids-1969-hiv-history-and-race/. Accessed 14 Mar 2020.

Kleinman, Arthur, and Joan Kleinman. 1997. The Appeal of Experience; The Dismay of Images: Cultural Appropriations of Suffering in Our Times. In *Social Suffering*, ed. Arthur Kleinman, Veena Das, and Margaret M. Lock, 1–23. Berkeley: University of California Press.

Kleinman, Arthur, Veena Das, and Margaret M. Lock. 1997. Introduction. In *Social Suffering*, ed. Arthur Kleinman, Veena Das, and Margaret M. Lock, ix–xxvii. Berkeley: University of California Press.

Mitchell, W.J. Thomas. 1994. *Picture Theory: Essays on Verbal and Visual Representation.* Chicago: University of Chicago Press.

Morris, David B. 1997. About Suffering: Voice, Genre, and Moral Community. In *Social Suffering*, ed. Arthur Kleinman, Veena Das, and Margaret M. Lock, 25–45. Berkeley: University of California Press.

O'Brian, Cormac. 2017. HIV and AIDS in Irish Theatre: Queer Masculinities, Punishment, and 'Post-AIDS' Culture. *Journal of Medical Humanities* 41: 123–136.

Patton, Cindy. 1990. *Inventing AIDS.* London: Routledge.

Redhead, Steve. 2008. *The Jean Baudrillard Reader.* Edinburgh: Edinburgh University Press.

Silverstone, Roger. 2004. The Sociology of Mediation and Communication. In *The SAGE Handbook of Sociological Analysis*, ed. Craig Calhoun, Chris Rojek, and Bryan Turner, 188–207. London: SAGE.

Singleton, Brian. 2011. *Masculinities and the Contemporary Irish Theatre.* Basingstoke: Palgrave Macmillan.

Sontag, Susan. 2003. *Regarding the Pain of Others.* New York: Farrar, Straus, and Giroux.

Watney, Simon. 1987. *Policing Desire: Pornography, AIDS, and the Media.* Minneapolis: University of Minnesota Press.

CHAPTER 3

#BeMoreJill and the Limited Visibility of Female Carers in *It's a Sin*

Janey Umback

3.1 Introduction

It's a Sin (2021) chronicles the lives of a group of young people coming of age during the first decade of the HIV/AIDS crisis in Britain, with five episodes set between 1981 and 1991. Focussing on friends and 'Pink Palace' housemates Ritchie Tozer (Olly Alexander), Roscoe Babatunde (Omari Douglas), Ash Mukherjee (Nathaniel Curtis), Colin Morris-Jones (Callum Scott Howells), and Jill Baxter (Lydia West), *It's a Sin* is described by series creator Russell T Davies as a story of "friends, lovers and families too—especially Jill, the girl who loves them and helps them, and galvanises them for the battles to come" (Subedar 2021). With this quote, Davies qualifies the character of Jill as a protector and as the programme's central uniting force.

J. Umback (✉)
Curtin University, Bentley, WA, Australia
e-mail: janey.umback@postgrad.curtin.edu.au

A. Castillo Villanueva, A. Bollas (eds.), *HIV/AIDS in Memory, Culture and Society*, Palgrave Studies in Science and Popular Culture, https://doi.org/10.1007/978-3-031-59699-5_3

It's a Sin carries with it aspects of modern LGBTQIA+[1] history and shares narratives relating to the HIV/AIDS epidemic that have, for the most part, been absent from mainstream media. Indeed, these aspects are only exacerbated by the viewing audience's awareness of the fraught historical context of the HIV/AIDS crisis in the United Kingdom during the 1980s and 1990s, including the introduction of Margaret Thatcher's Section 28 clause—a law prohibiting the promotion of homosexuality by local authorities including schools, radio, newspapers, and television. With this context, *It's a Sin* provides its viewers with access to stories from the front lines of the HIV/AIDS crisis that have not previously been broadcast on mainstream television.

Promotion during the broadcast of the series on Chanel 4 in the United Kingdom paid particular attention to Davies' 'real-life' connections to many of the characters portrayed on the screen. Notably, Davies' childhood friend Jill Nalder, an actor and prolific HIV/AIDS activist, was recognised as the inspiration behind the creation of the series and the character of 'Jill'. Summarising the series, the *BBC* noted, "Jill Nalder, who lost three friends to Aids in the 1980s, remembers how young men who contracted the virus at the time would 'disappear'" (Lawthom 2021, emphasis in original). In its review of the series, *Radio Times* stated, "Davies also based an *It's a Sin* character, Jill Baxter on a real-life 'inspiring' person from the period" (Carr 2021, emphasis in original). As part of an interview with Jill Nalder in the lead up to the release of *It's a Sin*, journalist Megan Sutton (2021) wrote for *Good Housekeeping Magazine*:

> Davies was inspired by his long-time friend Jill Nalder when writing the drama and in the show, Jill Baxter (played by Lydia West) is a character drawn from the life she's led ... Jill, now 60, lived in London in the '80s in the actual Pink Palace (a key setting in *It's a Sin*) and supported many gay men affected by the AIDS crisis.

These reviews provide some context for the development of the limited series and highlight the vital role that Jill Nalder played as a caregiver to people living with HIV/AIDS in the United Kingdom in the 1980s and 1990s.

[1] This chapter applies the acronym 'LGBTQIA+' to represent lesbian, gay, bisexual, transgender, intersex, queer/questioning, asexual/ally, and an evolving spectrum of terms (such as non-binary and pansexual) that people may use to describe their experiences of their gender, sexuality, and physiological sex characteristics.

Depicted by the BAFTA-nominated Lydia West, the character of Jill Baxter provides insight into the experience of female carers during a time in history when HIV/AIDS was primarily classified as a "gay man's disease" (Watney 1987). Emerging as a staunch activist and advocate across the five episodes of *It's a Sin*, Jill remains a loyal ally to her close-knit group of male friends as they each individually come to terms with the realities of the HIV/AIDS crisis. Yet, despite the publicity surrounding the influence of Jill Nalder and the incorporation of her 'real-life' experiences within the series, several media critics note the character's lack of personal development. For example, in its review of *It's a Sin*, *The British Film Industry* laments that Jill "is too defined by her relationship to the men in the story" (Davidson 2021), while entertainment website *Vulture* writes, "characters like Roscoe and Jill are so frustrating—the series does not care enough about exploring their inner lives or letting them share the spotlight" (VanArendonk 2021). Media critic Richard Lawson (2021) also summarises the dichotomy of Jill and *It's a Sin* for *Vanity Fair* magazine, suggesting that the character is the one "constant" throughout the story. However, Jill remains "underserved by her vagueness" (Lawson 2021) and is not given a purpose beyond her involvement in mutual aid and activism.

Using the publicity surrounding Jill Nalder as an example, this chapter suggests that the lack of character development for Jill Baxter in *It's a Sin* is indicative of the invisible work that female caregivers carried out during the first decade of the HIV/AIDS crisis in the global North. While many women took on caregiving roles for their HIV-positive friends and family members in the decade that *It's a Sin* is situated in (1981–1991), like Jill, their stories are rarely documented; when they are, they are reduced to 'supporting' characters. Setting this analysis in dialogue with existing scholarship of depictions of HIV/AIDS on popular television, this chapter begins with an introduction to the character of Jill Baxter, providing an overview of her role as a caregiver to the characters of Ritchie and Colin (amongst others). The chapter then discusses the representation of caregiving in *It's a Sin* to detail how popular television not only shapes perceptions but also changes viewers' memories of the HIV/AIDS crisis. This chapter closes with an examination of the hashtag #BeMoreJill that outlines how the hashtag became a platform encouraging second-screen viewing, bringing members of *It's a Sin's* viewing audience together to share their stories of HIV/AIDS allyship and advocacy.

3.2 Caregiving for People with HIV/AIDS

Given the substantial success of *It's a Sin*, this chapter offers a consideration of the breakout character of Jill Baxter as an ally and advocate on and off screen. First, as a loyal ally to Ritchie, Roscoe, Ash, and Colin, Jill provides significant comfort and leadership. Off screen, the lack of character development for Jill Baxter facilitates important conversations surrounding the lack of visibility for caregivers during the first decade of the HIV/AIDS crisis. This chapter suggests that opportunities need to be created that increase the visibility of (often unpaid) caregivers. An increase in visibility for caregivers, including more nuanced depictions of caregiving characters in film and on television, would allow their contributions to be granted proper acknowledgement by other members of their communities, including governments and policymakers.

Several community-based organisations, including the Gay Men's Health Crisis (GMHC), a North American non-profit organisation dedicated to serving members of the queer community, became high-profile organisations that provided care for HIV/AIDS positive individuals during the mid-1980s and into the 1990s. However, daily caregiving work remained a somewhat invisible task during this era. During the first decade of the HIV/AIDS crisis, caregiving for people with HIV/AIDS was a private, intimate act that was most often confined to domestic environments due to the high levels of stigma associated with the virus (Klassen 2021; Noe 2019). Contemporary research indicates that up to 90% of palliative care, including care for people with HIV/AIDS, still takes place at home (WHO 2023). This research also suggests that it is most often female caregivers who shoulder the greatest amount of responsibility for the physical and emotional care of family, friends, and community members with HIV/AIDS. It is not unusual for these generally unpaid, predominantly female caregivers to structure their caregiving responsibilities around hours of paid employment, as well as subsidising their caregiving with their own energy, time, and resources.

As HIV/AIDS caregiving has been subject to only a limited amount of academic attention, this analysis draws from a very small body of research. To date, accounts of HIV/AIDS caregiving in the global North mostly describe LGBTQIA+ community responses to the crisis. For example, in her book *Globalizing AIDS* (2002), sociologist Cindy Patton moves to classify the caregiving that took place during the first decade of the HIV/AIDS crisis as a form of AIDS activism. Patton notes that the caregiving responses by individuals and their personal and social networks helped facilitate the development of organisational infrastructure (2002, xvii), a necessary requirement for the development of activist-oriented responses to the crisis. More recently, Catungal et al. (2021) suggest that the majority of activist responses to the HIV/AIDS crisis prioritised the experiences of white, higher-income, gay men. Their argument indicates that many of the predominant narratives surrounding HIV/AIDS that emerged in the 1980s and 1990s have had long-term, at times negative, impacts resulting from segregating HIV/AIDS care and community work along racial, class, and geographic lines. They apply oral history narratives from long-term survivors of HIV/AIDS to discuss a number of intersectional exclusions and community practices that came to be associated with HIV/AIDS care provision and community-building efforts during the first decade of the crisis. Catungal et al.'s (2021) research stresses the limitations of the, at times, simplistic and often celebratory narratives that accompany much of the literature regarding early mobilisations in response to HIV/AIDS. Their work implies that female caregivers, in particular, have been provided with limited opportunities to share stories of their personal experiences. Their findings highlight the lack of representation for female caregivers during the first decade of the HIV/AIDS crisis, which could very easily be applied to the character of Jill Baxter.

3.3 Knowing Jill Baxter

As the female lead on *It's a Sin*, Jill Baxter quickly endears herself as "the unifying force and beating heart of the show" (Hattenstone 2021), simultaneously emerging as a mother figure, protector, cheerleader, and spiritual guide. In an interview with *Bustle* magazine, actor Lydia West described Jill as "driven from a place of love and care" (Jana 2021). Through compassion and humour, Jill enables her male friends to confront their deepest fears and feelings. Developing a particularly close bond with Ritchie Tozer, Jill becomes a mentor, arming him with the courage to follow his passion for acting, as well as facilitating the 'coming out' process with his family. Yet, despite her character's significance, and unlike Ritchie, Roscoe, and Colin's, Jill's personal life remains conspicuously underexplored within the limited television series. Instead, her storyline operates as a nexus to connect the male leads and share their narratives in depth. Jill's first appearance on screen sees her playing the role of Cupid, setting up university friend Ash with new student Ritchie. While Ash and

Ritchie's romance is short-lived, the 'meet cute' that occurs between Jill and Ritchie is the thread tying the lead characters together. Jill, who the viewing audience learns is an aspiring actor, evolves throughout the narrative of *It's a Sin*. She is first introduced as the supportive best friend before shifting into the roles of caregiver, urgent activist, and, finally, the mouthpiece for *It's a Sin*'s final heart-wrenching monologue. With her closing words, Jill unloads the burden of being the lead character through which the limited television series' messages of compassion and advocacy are hung.

In his interview with *Damian Barr's Literary Salon* (2021), Russell T Davies explains how he had originally planned for eight episodes of the historical drama, including a flash forward to Jill's life set 30 years in the future. He shares, "she's still working in mental and sexual health. It's too long a story to describe, but you get the feeling that she's trapped in that world actually" (Barr 2021) Within the same interview, Davies details how the viewing audience would have seen Jill "going on cruise ships and to conference centres and singing songs in the West End with all her mates" (Barr 2021). These episodes were cut from the final script, although Davies made a point to share that they had been budgeted for in the lead-up to production. In his review of *It's a Sin*, journalist Tim Murphy (2021) expresses his disappointment that the viewing audience was not able to experience a well-rounded Baxter. Murphy observes how Jill Nalder's brief cameo as Jill's own mother is one of the few times "we learn anything about Jill outside of her role as Florence Nightingale to gay men" (Murphy 2021). Without the backstory that Davies had planned out initially, it is impossible to conceptualise any aspect of the character outside of her relationships with her housemates. As Murphy (2021) continues,

> we don't know if she likes boys, girls, or both; we don't know how she feels about being biracial amid the racial complexities of her friend group; we don't know if she has any ambivalence about her role as decade-long, 24-7 angel of mercy and de facto case manager for all her friends; and we get no intimation whether, or how, the tremendous emotional and logistical toll this young woman is under will affect her the rest of her life.

What is particularly clear is that the absence of a fully developed storyline for Jill echoes the absence of mainstream narratives relating to female carers during the first decade of the HIV/AIDS crisis in the global North. While LGBTQIA+ communities struggled to come to terms with the trauma, grief, and homophobia associated with HIV/AIDS, groups of women stood up to take care of their friends and loved ones while hospitals and doctors refused to see them due to the introduction of Section 28 and the dissemination/proliferation of harmful myths surrounding the virus (Noe 2019).

Activism and advocacy relating to the provision of health care have been a pivotal facet of feminist engagement since the emergence of the women's rights movement in the 1960s (Morgen 2002). It is notable, then, that during the first decade of the HIV/AIDS crisis, gay men were subject to the poignant teachings that the women's rights movement had been articulating and documenting for decades. Faced with the exigencies of HIV/AIDS, gay men found themselves needing to navigate the medical establishment by openly identifying as 'men who have sex with men' (Anderson 1998; Ross 1989; Warwick et al. 2001), only to be subject to the biases, neglect, and ignorance that resonated strongly with the experiences of women. The hierarchical frameworks of the medical establishment, as well as the ideological objectives of scientific medicine in the global North, and the vulnerability of marginalised social groups all became important topics of discussion during this time. Yet, this does not mean to imply that women's requirements concerning HIV/AIDS received distinctive or superior consideration; rather, that male homosexuality became assimilated into the disease paradigm for HIV/AIDS, resulting in the substantial oversight of women in this context.

In her discussion of issues relating to women's experiences of HIV/AIDS, sociologist Diane Richardson (1996) highlights a lack of research relating to women's experiences during the first decade of the HIV/AIDS crisis. She suggests that in the United Kingdom, the geographical location of *It's a Sin*, the experiences of women have been greatly repressed. Richardson categorises the lack of representation for women as a "male-ing of AIDS" (1996, 163) that continues to impact public understandings of the virus—from the broad public denial that women are at risk of contracting HIV/AIDS, through to male-only samples being used to trial HIV/AIDS medications. Richardson's work suggests that women in HIV/AIDS-related media discourse are portrayed as either the wives of HIV-positive men who have had extramarital affairs or the mothers of HIV-positive children. In some media representations, as occurs within the plot of *It's a Sin*, women may fall into the character trope of mothers who 'fail' in their maternal caregiving duties by rejecting their HIV-positive children (Richardson 1996, 165). However, it has also been suggested that in many 'real-life' scenarios, women are highly likely to experience stigma from family members, neighbours, and their communities if they maintain close physical contact with an HIV-positive spouse or child (Ogden and Nyblade 2005; Deacon 2006). While these findings do not attempt to excuse this behaviour, they indicate a lack of nuance for female characters in many HIV/AIDS media narratives.

There are problems with representation in programmes like *It's a Sin* that should be addressed in order for women to have their stories and experiences shared with an appropriate amount of detail. As visibility has undoubtedly increased for members of LGBTQIA+ communities, one can only remain hopeful that visibility for women, particularly those in caregiving roles, will follow in their wake. As feminist scholar Paula Treichler argues, "the AIDS epidemic poses problems of representation, identity, and narrative conventions for network television" (1999, 176). In this case, television series' contributions towards giving visibility to characters like Jill Baxter need to be addressed in order to add personal meaning and nuance to their lives. Increased visibility for both women and caregivers provides many noteworthy rewards. These rewards include greater social recognition and a reduction of potentially harmful stereotypes.

3.4 Female Caregiving and 'Doing Gender' in *It's a Sin*

Over the course of five episodes, *It's a Sin* chronicles how a group of friends, predominantly from LGBTQIA+ and minoritised ethnic communities, confront the toll of HIV/AIDS. Cementing the idea that shame, marginalisation, and the lack of media representation were the key drivers making the first decade of the HIV/AIDS epidemic so devastating, the programme's plotline builds towards a powerful closing statement by Jill Baxter. It has become clear over the course of the series that Baxter's best friend, series protagonist Ritchie, has been raised by his parents to feel ashamed of his identity. This shame, coupled with a sense that his life as a gay male is an embarrassment, is indicative of the behaviours that fuelled the spread of the virus. As Jill reflects to Ritchie's mother, Valerie Tozer (Keeley Hawes) in the final episode of *It's a Sin*,

> The wards are full of men who think they deserve it. They are dying, and a little bit of them thinks, *yes, this is right. I brought this on myself; it's my fault* (emphasis added).

The marginalisation of members of the queer community in the global North, as well as a mainstream refusal to view queer lives as valuable, was foundational to the devastating spread of HIV/AIDS. *It's a Sin* reconceptualises this notion by advocating for a generation of young individuals abandoned by their families, through emphasising the importance of chosen rather than biological family. Families, biological or otherwise, are predominantly observed through gendered expectations of behaviours. Sociologists Candace West and Donald Zimmerman (1987)[2] describe gender as a routine aspect of our everyday lives that is reinforced through institutional and social interactions (1987, 137). They consider gender to be a social construction and note that 'doing gender' is "unavoidable" as long as "society is partitioned by 'essential' differences between women and men" (West and Zimmerman 1987, 137). This means that they see gender as not what a person is but rather the ways that a person acts during their social interactions with others. To apply West and Zimmerman's concept of 'doing gender' to *It's a Sin,* we could say that when Jill participates in acts of caregiving, she is fulfilling a role that is predominantly associated with being female. The type of caregiving work that Jill participates in, including aiding with daily living activities, such as bathing and dressing, as well as contributory activities, including shopping, cooking, and cleaning, are most regularly conflated with women's labour. *It's a Sin* devotes much screentime to highlighting the ways that Jill cares for several friends as they individually face their own battles with HIV/

[2] The choice to integrate West and Zimmerman's concept of 'doing gender' (1987) within this chapter, rather than applying Judith Butler's concepts of gender performativity (1990, 1993) has come down to the specific context of *It's a Sin*. Both West and Zimmerman, as well as Butler, have made significant contributions to the understanding of gender, but they approach the concept from two unique perspectives. West and Zimmerman's 'doing gender' theory focuses on the idea that gender is not simply a fixed identity or role but is actively accomplished through everyday interactions. They emphasise that individuals engage in 'doing gender' through their behaviours, actions, and performances, reinforcing societal expectations and norms related to gender—in this case, the way that the character of Jill Baxter is primarily depicted in the traditionally 'feminine' role of primary caregiver in *It's a Sin*. Judith Butler challenges the idea that gender is a stable identity and argues that it is a repeated performance, enacted through speech, gestures, and other behaviours. Butler's work provides insights into power dynamics and the agentic behaviours of individuals to resist or subvert normative gender performances, yet this chapter does not read this as characteristic of the actions of Jill Baxter within the five episodes of *It's a Sin*. However, this chapter recognises that West and Zimmerman's 'doing gender' and Butler's gender performativity are not mutually exclusive. These concepts complement each other and increase our understanding of the complexities of gender within our daily interactions.

AIDS. Throughout this process, the viewing audience bears witness to Jill providing (unpaid) caregiving acts such as cooking, cleaning, and further educating herself in an effort to keep her friends protected. Despite the complex narrative canvas displayed within *It's a Sin*, one aspect deserving more critical examination is the conspicuously limited character development of Jill. The series, while weaving a rich tapestry of interconnected lives, regrettably falls short when illustrating the nuanced dimensions of Jill's self-care. Rather than developing her personal journey and the ways in which she tends to her own needs, the narrative remains predominantly fixated on the arcs of its male characters. This inadvertent neglect of Jill not only obscures her individual growth but also raises questions about the series' broader thematic priorities, prompting a closer examination of the underlying dynamics that shape the portrayal of its central characters.

As the series progresses, Jill becomes more outspoken, arranging protests and volunteering in call centres and hospitals. Viewers can only assume that Jill provides this labour outside of regular working hours, as there is no mention of how her lifestyle is maintained or what her lifestyle involves beyond the scope of providing for her friend's wellbeing. It remains unknown how Jill can find balance in performing multiple duties and facing the emotional and physical toll of caregiving and losing friends. However, her increased responsibilities are on par with the expectations that have been set through the ways that Jill 'does gender' (West and Zimmerman 1987). With much of the promotion of *It's a Sin* built around the importance of Jill, it seems a shame that she is not given adequate character development outside the undoubtedly valuable role of caring for her friends. As journalist Madeline Ducharme (2021) reiterates for *SLATE* magazine, "Jill deserved a life beyond caring for the boys." Similarly, in response to the series, AIDS activist and author Victoria Noe states in conversation with journalist Tim Murphy (2021),

> I wanted to say to Jill, "Get out of there now—just stop!" She paid the price for everybody. She kept their secrets. She did everything for them, including trying to educate them, which they did not appreciate at all [at first].[3] She loved them and took care of them, even when she knew they were doing things that would hurt them. They let her do everything for them. It was very rare in the series for one of the guys to say to her, "Can I go with you?"

[3] The information provided within the square brackets of this quote is provided within this article by Tim Murphy (2021).

> [to the hospital or an AIDS-related obligation]. And she had this supposedly wonderful job—as an actress—that you see for five seconds in five hours. She doesn't have a life. Nobody ever asks Jill, "Are you OK?"

Television is considered a primary medium through which predominantly heteronormative values are regularly shared. The presence of a 'heterosexual script' (Kim et al. 2007; Seabrook et al. 2016) on popular television helps define viewers' understandings of sex while also providing direction on how to recognise romantic and sexual situations. Kim et al. (2007) identify the presence of a dominant 'heterosexual script' that comprises corresponding scripts guiding men and women during romantic and sexual interactions. In the heterosexual script, men are assumed to prioritise sex over relationships. On the other hand, women are portrayed as sexually passive, prioritising romantic relationships over sex. Consequently, the presence of a 'heterosexual script' and the lack of development for characters like Jill on popular television are notable points that should be addressed in narratives relating to HIV/AIDS. But, as Noe (2019) outlines, the indelible and excessive absence of women's stories in media portrayals of HIV/AIDS is unfortunately on par with the lack of resources that describe the reality of women's contributions to HIV/AIDS research, advocacy, care, and education—both within and beyond the LGBTQIA+ communities that are most commonly associated with the virus.

3.5 Those Left Behind: *It's a Sin* and Visibility on Popular Television

It's a Sin should be commended for its contribution towards increasing awareness of the impact of the HIV/AIDS crisis on members of LGBTQIA+ communities during the 1980s and 1990s. The portrayal of HIV-positive characters in the programme as active, vibrant, fun, and loving manifests a prevailing need to replace dominant popular cultural discourses with more 'realistic' portrayals of members of LGBTQIA+ communities during a time when HIV/AIDS became an ever-present reality. While many of the scenes in *It's a Sin* are imbued with tragedy, the limited television series is also laced with funny and often charming moments. Notably, in the first episode, the three intersecting storylines that result in Ritchie, Roscoe, and Colin establishing roots in London are filled with youthful exuberance. The opening scenes of *It's a Sin* are hopeful, illustrating how these three young men are liberated through establishing community, sexual experimentation, and becoming loved for who they genuinely are. Communication scholar Malynnda Johnson (2013) suggests that the use of HIV/AIDS narratives within popular media texts, including TV series, has a significant impact on viewers' perceptions of the virus (Johnson 2013, 1117). However, in her analysis of HIV/AIDS narratives in popular media texts, Johnson (2013) also makes note that for many viewers, HIV infection is perceived to occur only in "forgotten or unfamiliar worlds" (2013, 1117). Her work states that the lack of diverse visibility in the mainstream media for members of LGBTQIA+ communities during the first decade of the AIDS crisis often resulted in misunderstandings and feelings of shame linked to the virus.

The 1980s and 1990s saw a lack of representation for members of LGBTQIA+ communities who were excluded from state recognition and policies, with any effort to increase visibility being met with increased stigmatisation (Brouwer 1998). As queer people were largely absent from media discourse across several popular television programmes at the time, HIV/AIDS was portrayed as impacting the lives of predominantly white, heteronormative characters. One of the first portrayals of HIV/AIDS on television occurred in December 1983 on an episode of North American hospital drama *St Elsewhere.* In the episode *Aids and Comfort*, a married politician presents to the fictional St. Eligius Hospital after being infected with HIV via an extramarital (heterosexual) affair. Other programmes from the decade shared more family-centric storylines, such as the made-for-television movies *Go Toward the Light* (1988) and *The Ryan White Story* (1989). The women in these storylines were always depicted as wives and mothers, setting the tone for this somewhat familiar narrative. Both *Go Toward the Light* and *The Ryan White Story* told the life stories of young haemophiliac boys infected with HIV/AIDS after receiving blood transfusions. These three examples show how mainstream media focussed on how HIV/AIDS affected 'typical' white, North American, suburban families and ignored the direct impact of HIV and AIDS on LGBTQIA+ people, women, and other members of minoritised communities.

Malynnda Johnson's (2013) analysis of HIV/AIDS narratives in the mainstream media indicates a steady decline in television storylines relating to the virus since the 1990s. Reaffirming Johnson's findings, Kagan (2018, 2) suggests that HIV/AIDS-related storylines began to disappear from popular media with the introduction of antiretroviral drugs (ARVs) in 1996. As people were increasingly able to seek treatment for—and live with—HIV, their stories became increasingly scarce. Kagan further highlights "significant exceptions" to this rule, including Russell T Davies' *Queer as Folk* (1999–2000), as well as the ground-breaking North American miniseries *Angels in America* (2003). The dearth of HIV/AIDS-related storylines on popular television in the global North has been correspondingly addressed by journalist Manuel Betancourt (2021), who wrote for *New York Magazine*'s entertainment news website *Vulture*:

> According to GLAAD, in the 2020–2021 TV season, of 1,063 regular and recurring characters tracked across broadcast, cable, and streaming, only three characters were living with HIV. All three were on the same show, FX's period drama *Pose* (emphasis in the original).

Both Betancourt (2021) and Kagan (2018) detail how HIV/AIDS-related narratives have become one of the "hallmarks of period storytelling" (Betancourt 2021). Kagan notes "a flourishing of archival projects, visual art retrospectives, prestige period TV dramas ... remakes, remounts and crosstextual adaptations of literary and performing art works from earlier in the pandemic" (Kagan 2018, 2). While some contemporary programmes, including Amazon Prime Video's *Transparent* (2014–2019), provide occasion for viewers to observe HIV-positive characters in more modern contexts (Strause 2016), most recent depictions of HIV/AIDS on popular television have been retro set in the early years of the crisis. This includes titles such as Ryan Murphy's *Pose* (2018–2021) and *It's a Sin*. Kagan proposes that the amount of 'retro' HIV/AIDS narratives on television over the past 5 years coincides with an increased cultural interest in "AIDS activist histories, AIDS art and the aesthetics of the crisis years (in fashion, design, hairstyles and so on)" (2018, 206). However, Kagan's work also implies that the retro lens that is most commonly applied to depictions of the virus on television facilitates ways of shining light on a range of non-heteronormative storylines and, therefore, increases visibility for LGBTQIA+ individuals who have long been absent from AIDS-related media discourse. Yet, within these storylines, women remain relegated to being portrayed in caregiving roles, such as wife and mother, that intersect with traditional concepts of femininity.

Betancourt (2021) and Kagan (2018) address the significance of the increased visibility on TV for members of LGBTQIA+ communities. However, with the notable exceptions of the trans-female characters portrayed in *Transparent* and *Pose*, who by their very existence are breaking heteronormative concepts of what it means to be a 'woman,' other female characters remain largely invisible, or otherwise reduced to traditional caregiving roles within HIV/AIDS-related storylines on television. This lack of representation and nuance for female characters is noteworthy as it draws attention to the deep-seated issues surrounding gender norms and representation in global television industries. Prior media analyses examining portrayals of women on primetime television indicate two distinct trends. First, women continually appear at a rate below their proportion of the global population. For example, during the 2019–2020 television season in North America, only 43% of characters in speaking roles were female (Lauzen 2020). Second, women are often restricted to a strict number of roles on television that highlight idealised standards of beauty and gender-stereotypic occupations and lifestyles, including portrayals of wives, mothers, and other caregiving-adjacent roles (Scharrer 2012).

3.6 The Affordances of Social Media Hashtags and #BeMoreJill

One way *It's a Sin* may have attempted to develop the character of Jill is by incorporating the hashtag #BeMoreJill into the programme's social media advertising campaign. *It's a Sin* launched in the United Kingdom on 22 January 2021 to overwhelmingly positive feedback from critics and viewers. Data released from Channel 4 in the United Kingdom indicates that the series attracted an average audience of 2.3m viewers per episode. The debut of *It's a Sin* was the biggest drama launch for Channel 4 in 3 years among young viewers (18.4% share of 16–34-year-old viewers), while the United Kingdom-based HIV and sexual health charity Terrence Higgins Trust reported that across the week of *It's a Sin*'s debut episode, over 17k orders of HIV tests were placed in the United Kingdom—this was over double the quantity ordered during the previous *National HIV Testing Week* (8.2k). The charity's data, shared by Channel 4, also shows that its helpline, which provides support and advice around HIV and sexual health, had a 30% increase in calls the day after the debut of *It's a Sin* (Channel 4 2023).

A week after the programme's debut, on 28 January 2021, Russell T Davies posted a public thank-you message to his personal Twitter account. The tweet by Davies read:

> Folks! I can't answer everyone's #ItsaSin messages, I'd disappear. But cast and crew are astonished and delighted by the reaction, we've never seen anything like it. Thank you! La #BeMoreJill.

First integrated into users' posts on Twitter, the micro-blogging platform that is now known as X, hashtags are now commonly integrated into users' posts across most social media platforms. Hashtags give emphasis to or otherwise clarify the meaning of a user's post. For instance, a user who wants to emphasise that their post relates to the topic of caregiving may incorporate the hashtag #caregiving within the description section of the associated post. Similarly, a user who wants to find posts that specifically discuss caregiving can conduct a search for that specific hashtag. Davies' incorporation of the hashtag #BeMoreJill became a secondary avenue for viewers to connect with the program as well as with each other through discussing their own personal experiences that echoed Jill's experiences. Once posted by Davies, the hashtag #BeMoreJill quickly became a platform for Twitter users to engage with each other while bonding over the emotional and historical aspects of the program. Predominantly, the posts, including #BeMoreJill, focussed on acts of caregiving for people living with or who had lost their lives to HIV/AIDS.

At the time of writing, Davies' original #BeMoreJill Tweet has amassed 1696k retweets and 38.2k likes (Davies 2021); however, instead of reposting, most users have interacted with Davies' statement by using #BeMoreJill to share and connect their own personal narratives. The popularity of #BeMoreJill highlights how on-screen hashtags facilitate brand-building for television programmes and their creators. At the same time, hashtags create a space for self-expression and foster community amongst a specific audience. In this example, the character of Jill Baxter, now materialised through the impactful hashtag #BeMoreJill, serves as a pivotal force in the realms of HIV/AIDS caregiving and awareness. In this iteration, Jill plays a central role in fostering connections among television viewers, providing a platform for them to unite and engage with the programme's content. Describing the viral popularity of #BeMoreJill, *Bustle* magazine remarked that the hashtag became a platform of advocacy, "with thousands sharing the stories of the Jills in their own lives" (Jana 2021). In the same article by *Bustle*, actor Lydia West explicated both the character of Jill and the viral hashtag as holding a "humanity that we can all connect to" before moving on to describe the importance of sharing admiration "for the people we care about" (Jana 2021). In these instances, the hashtag #BeMoreJill becomes an excellent example of how the affordances of social media may increase visibility for caregivers.

In the field of Internet studies, the word 'affordances' is regularly used to discuss the relationships that are fostered between users, user behaviour, and digital technologies (Leonardi and Treem 2020). Affordances are interactive and are born from specific online contexts. For example, numerous people have the opportunity to interact with #BeMoreJill on Twitter; however, each user has the opportunity to add their own personal narratives to the hashtag. Affordances, such as the anonymity of a user or a user's visibility, are not features of the technology that they are engaging with. Rather, affordances are the perceived abilities of digital technologies to either assist or restrain behavioural outcomes. In discussions of social networking platforms such as Twitter, it is important to understand that it is the unique features of a platform (such as the incorporation of hashtags into the platform's interface) that facilitate a range of affordances for users. The affordances facilitated via hashtags like #BeMoreJill include increased visibility and association for users, bonding them together through feelings of community and shared experiences (Leonardi and Treem 2020).

Hashtags serve viewing audiences as facilitators of conversation and connection. However, the popularity of 'official' hashtags related to television programmes since 2011 has also been considered a strategic effort by television networks to utilise the temporal engagement of viewers to maximise profit and marketing reach (Proulx and Shepatin 2012). Television networks increasingly turn to social media to gauge viewers' reactions to their programs. This is because social media acts as "a giant unfiltered focus group" (Proulx and Shepatin 2012, 30), where viewers have the space to share their thoughts and opinions on a program. Proulx and Shepatin (2012) note that watching television has always been a social activity. However, social media provides easy ways for viewers to interact and converse with each other. Viewers have always discussed the television programmes that resonate with them, and hashtags have become an effective way to magnify viewers' conversations. It has become increasingly common for television programmes to produce official hashtags as a way of engaging audiences and encouraging interaction via 'second-screen' tweeting.

Second-screen tweeting is the result of an audience watching a programme while simultaneously keeping abreast of key trends and topics being discussed on social media. While television was once the key source of household entertainment, viewers' attention span is now spread across multiple screens and devices. Second-screen tweeting encourages viewers to stay abreast of a programme by encouraging FOMO (fear of missing out) while also holding attention across several devices. Beyond this more mainstream use of hashtags to encourage audience participation during a programme's broadcast, television shows that may appeal to more niche audiences, such as *It's a Sin*, may utilise official hashtags to engage with a more diverse community of viewers and increase their program's viewership. Hashtags operate as a tool that aids in the development of online communities; they can increase visibility and enable niche communities to be found and easily joined. However, the hashtag #BeMoreJill and the ways that users engage with it illustrate how the characterisation of Jill facilitates avenues of conversation regarding the invisibility of female caregivers in HIV/AIDS-related media contexts. The adoption of #BeMoreJill by viewers of *It's a Sin* creates an avenue to increase visibility for 'real-life Jills'. Utilising the hashtag, users shared stories and images of the valuable women in their lives, while others incorporated #BeMoreJill to promote HIV/AIDS education and awareness.

3.7 Conclusion

Using the publicity surrounding Jill Nalder as an example, this chapter has suggested that the lack of character development for Jill Baxter in *It's a Sin* is indicative of the invisible work that female caregivers carried out during the first decade of the HIV/AIDS crisis. While many women took on caregiving roles for their HIV-positive friends and family members throughout the decade that *It's a Sin* is situated in (1981–1991), like Jill, their stories are rarely broadcast, or they have likewise been reduced to 'supporting' characters. By setting this analysis in dialogue with existing scholarship of depictions of HIV/AIDS on popular television, this chapter provided an overview of Jill Baxter's role as a caregiver to the characters of Ritchie and Colin, amongst others. This chapter then discussed the representation of caregiving on *It's a Sin* to detail how popular television shapes viewers' perceptions of HIV/AIDS.

Given the substantial success of *It's a Sin*, this chapter considers the breakout character of Jill Baxter as an ally and advocate on and off screen. First, as a loyal ally to Ritchie, Roscoe, Ash, and Colin, Jill provides significant comfort and leadership. Off screen, the lack of character development for Jill Baxter has facilitated important conversations surrounding the lack of visibility for caregivers during the first decade of the HIV/AIDS crisis.

This chapter has suggested that opportunities must be created that increase the visibility of often unpaid, often female caregivers. An increase in visibility for caregivers, including more nuanced depictions of caregiving characters in film and on television, would allow their contributions to be granted proper acknowledgement by other members of their communities, including governments and policymakers. While this chapter has noted that much has been gained in terms of the recognition of LGBTQIA+ communities during the first decade of the HIV/AIDS crisis in the global North, there remains a distinct lack of visibility for female caregivers. Furthermore, while the integration of Jill Nalder's story into the promotional campaign for *It's a Sin*, along with #BeMoreJill, may facilitate an increase in visibility for female caregivers, this community requires more critical media intervention to further assist the sharing of female caregiver's stories.

References

Anderson, Andrew L. 1998. Strengths of Gay Male Youth: An Untold Story. *Child and Adolescent Social Work Journal* 15: 55–71.

Barr, Damien. 2021. Salon on Demand: Russell T Davies & Ruth Coker Burks with Damian Barr. *Damian Barr's Literary Salon*, February 18. https://www.damianbarr.com/events/2021/2/19/salon-on-demand-russell-t-davies-ruth-coker-burks-with-with-damian-barr. Accessed 2 June 2022.

Betancourt, Manuel. 2021. How TV Stories Have Shaped Our Understanding of AIDS. *Vulture*, February 25. https://www.vulture.com/article/tv-aids-hiv-television-story-timeline.html. Accessed 1 June 2022.

Brouwer, Dan. 1998. The Precarious Visibility Politics of Self-Stigmatization: The Case of HIV/AIDS Tattoos. *Text and Performance Quarterly* 18: 114–136. https://doi.org/10.1080/10462939809366216. Accessed 10 Dec 2023.

Butler, Judith. 1993. *Bodies That Matter*. New York: Routledge.

———. 1990. *Gender Trouble*. New York: Routledge.

Catungal, John Paul, Benjamin Klassen, Robert Ablenas, Sandy Lambert, Sarah Chown, and Nathan Lachowsky. 2021. Organising Care and Community in the Era of the 'Gay Disease': Gay Community Responses to HIV/AIDS and the Production of Differentiated Care Geographies in Vancouver. *Urban Studies* 58 (7): 1346–1363.

Carr, Flora. 2021. The Real-Life History Behind Channel 4 Drama It's a Sin. *Radio Times*, January 22. https://www.radiotimes.com/tv/drama/its-a-sin-real-life-history-hiv-aids/. Accessed 1 June 2022.

Channel 4. 2023. Channel 4's It's a Sin Hits 18.9m All 4 Views and Helps Drive Increase in HIV Testing. *4Sales*. https://www.4sales.com/latest/2021-03/news/channel-4s-its-sin-hits-189m-all-4-views-and-helps-drive-increase-hiv-testing#:~:text=Viewing%20figures%20released%20today%20along,m%20views%20on%20All%204*. Accessed 10 Dec 2023.

Davidson, Alex. 2021. It's a Sin Is a Love Letter to 1980s Gay Culture—and Hate Mail to the Era's Homophobic Hegemony. *BFI*, January 22. https://www.bfi.org.uk/sight-and-sound/reviews/its-sin-russell-t-davies-channel-4-aids-drama-series-1980s-gay-culture. Accessed 2 June 2022.

Davies, Russell T. 2021. Folks! *Twitter*, January 28. https://twitter.com/russelldavies63/status/1354817622269808653?ref_src=twsrc%5Etfw%7Ctwcamp%5Etweetembed%7Ctwterm%5E1354817622269808653%7Ctwgr%5E%7Ctwcon%5Es1_&ref_url=https%3A%2F%2Fwww.pinknews.co.uk%2F2021%2F01%2F29%2Fits-a-sin-russell-t-davies-fan-reaction-be-more-jill-lgbt%2F. Accessed 1 May 2022.

Deacon, Harriett. 2006. Towards a Sustainable Theory of Health-Related Stigma: Lessons from the HIV/AIDS Literature. *Journal of Community & Applied Social Psychology* 16 (6): 418–425. https://onlinelibrary.wiley.com/doi/pdfdirect/10.1002/casp.900?casa_token=vLtGv-cMvgsAAAAA:8umtu1YqjQGQa6FVbSoajx0vlZkknCzLjDtI6GiJnAUvXoznL7TxC-erXNOI9ruPGBLl6dl6OtorKK1SbA. Accessed 5 Nov 2023.

Ducharme, Madeline. 2021. *It's a Sin* Failed to Give Women Their Rightful Place in the AIDS Story. *SLATE Magazine*, March 4. https://slate.com/culture/2021/03/its-a-sin-aids-hbo-jill.html. Accessed 1 May 2022.

Hattenstone, Simon. 2021. Interview: Russell T Davies: 'I Genuinely Thought, Who Wants to Watch a Show about AIDS?'. *The Guardian*, December 22. https://www.theguardian.com/tv-and-radio/2021/dec/22/russell-t-davies-i-genuinely-thought-who-wants-to-watch-a-show-about-aids. Accessed 1 June 2022.

Jana, Rosalind. 2021. Lydia West Will Never Say Goodbye to Jill, Not Really. *Bustle*, March 3. https://www.bustle.com/entertainment/lydia-west-talks-its-a-sin-bemorejill-cut-storylines. Accessed 1 May 2022.

Johnson, Malynnda. 2013. More Than Pop Culture: Depictions of HIV in the Media and the Effect on Viewer's Perception of Risk. *Journal of Homosexuality* 60 (8): 1117–1142. https://doi.org/10.1080/00918369.2013.776423. Accessed 5 November 2023.

Kagan, Dion. 2018. *Positive Images: Gay Men and HIV/AIDS in the Culture of 'Post-Crisis'*. London: I.B Tauris.

Kim, Janna L., C. Lynn Sorsoli, Katherine Collins, Bonnie A. Zylbergold, Deborah Schooler, and Deborah L. Tolman. 2007. From Sex to Sexuality: Exposing the Heterosexual Script on Primetime Network Television. *Journal of Sex Research* 44 (2): 145–157.

Klassen, Benjamin. 2021. Facing It Together: Early Caregiving Responses to Vancouver's HIV/AIDS Epidemic. *Gender & History* 33 (3): 774–789.

Lauzen, Martha M. 2020. Boxed in 2019-20: Women on Screen and Behind the Scenes in Television. *Women in TV and Film*. https://womenintvfilm.sdsu.edu/wp-content/uploads/2020/09/2019-2020_Boxed_In_Report.pdf. Accessed 5 Nov 2023.

Lawson, Richard. 2021. *It's a Sin* Is an Affecting AIDS Drama, but an Incomplete History. *Vanity Fair*, February 17. https://www.vanityfair.com/hollywood/2021/02/review-its-a-sin-is-an-affecting-aids-drama-but-an-incomplete-history. Accessed 1 May 2022.

Lawthom, Jared. 2021. It's A Sin: The Woman Who Inspired Russell T Davies' Aids Drama. *BBC News*, February 5. https://www.bbc.com/news/uk-wales-55937944. Accessed 5 November 2023.

Leonardi, Paul M., and Jeffrey W. Treem. 2020. Behavioral Visibility: A New Paradigm for Organization Studies in the Age of Digitization, Digitalization, and Datafication. *Organization Studies* 41 (12): 1601–1625. https://doi.org/10.1177/0170840620970728. Accessed 5 Nov 2023.

Morgen, Sandra. 2002. *Into Our Own Hands: The Women's Health Movement in the United States, 1969-1990*. New Brunswick: Rutgers University Press.

Murphy, Tim. 2021. What is The Inner Life of Jill Baxter on 'It's A Sin'? *The Body*, March 11. https://www.thebody.com/article/jill-baxter-its-a-sin. Accessed 30 May 2022.

Noe, Victoria. 2019. *F*g Hags, Divas and Moms: The Legacy of Straight Women in the AIDS Community*. Chicago: King Company Publishing.

Ogden, Jessica, and Laura Nyblade. 2005. *Common at Its Core: HIV-Related Stigma Across Contexts*, 1–45. International Center for Research on Women. https://www.icrw.org/publications/common-at-its-core-hiv-related-stigma-across-contexts/. Accessed 5 Nov 2023.

Patton, Cindy. 2002. *Globalizing AIDS*. Minneapolis: University of Minnesota Press.

Proulx, Mike, and Stacey Shepatin. 2012. *Social TV: How Marketers Can Reach and Engage Audiences by Connecting Television to the Web, Social Media, and Mobile*. Hoboken: Wiley.

Richardson, Diane. 1996. *Women and the AIDS Crisis*. London: Rivers Oram Press/Pandora List.

Ross, Michael W. 1989. Gay Youth in Four Cultures: A Comparative Study. *Journal of Homosexuality* 17: 299–314.

Seabrook, Rita C., L. Monique Ward, Lauren Reed, Adriana Manago, Soraya Giaccardi, and Julia R. Lippman. 2016. Our Scripted Sexuality: The Development and Validation of a Measure of the Heterosexual Script and Its Relation to Television Consumption. *Emerging Adulthood* 4 (5): 338–355.

Scharrer, Erica. 2012. More Than "Just the Facts"?: Portrayals of Masculinity in Police and Detective Programs Over Time. *Howard Journal of Communications* 23 (1): 88–109.

Strause, Jackie. 2016. 'Transparent' Star on Josh and Shea's Ground-breaking Romance: 'It's Just Boy Meets Girl'. *Hollywood Reporter*, October 4. https://www.hollywoodreporter.com/tv/tv-news/transparents-josh-shea-trace-lysette-934860/#. Accessed 31 May 2022.

Subedar, Anisa. 2021. It's A Sin: The Real Women Who Cared. *BBC News*, February 19. https://www.bbc.com/news/uk-55928870. Accessed 1 June 2022.

Sutton, Megan. 2021. It's A Sin's Jill Nalder: Meet the Woman Whose Real Life Inspired the Hit Drama. *Good Housekeeping*, February 5. https://www.goodhousekeeping.com/uk/lifestyle/a35419173/its-a-sin-jill-nalder-interview/. Accessed 2 June 2022.

Treichler, Paula A. 1999. *How to Have Theory in an Epidemic: Cultural Chronicles of AIDS*. Durham: Duke University Press.

VanArendonk, Kathryn. 2021. *It's a Sin*'s Clear-Eyed Look at the AIDS Crisis Has One Big Blind Spot. *Vulture*, February 18. https://www.vulture.com/article/its-a-sin-review-hbo-max.html. Accessed 1 May 2022.

Warwick, Ian, Peter Aggleton, and Nicola Douglas. 2001. Playing It Safe: Addressing the Emotional and Physical Health of Lesbian and Gay Pupils in the UK. *Journal of Adolescence* 24 (1): 129–140.

Watney, Simon. 1987. People's Perceptions of the Risk of Aids and the Role of the Mass Media. *Health Education Journal* 46 (2): 62–65. https://journals.sagepub.com/doi/pdf/10.1177/001789698704600209?casa_token=4AAIzy36oSsAAAAA:lqNTOQyGH-6X7qOnth7ssh5LPquyuZa6cNflkoD72auKC2Aw_K24qBFyUmmbI6ECaKxPMKrwS_Zdeho. Accessed 4 Nov 2023.

West, Candace, and Donald H. Zimmerman. 1987. Doing Gender. *Gender & Society* 1 (2): 125–151. https://doi.org/10.1177/0891243287001002002. Accessed 5 November 2023.

World Health Organization (WHO). 2023. HIV and AIDS, July 13. https://www.who.int/news-room/fact-sheets/detail/hiv-aids. Accessed 5 Nov 2023.

List of Television Programs

Herzfeld, John. 1989. *The Ryan White Story*, January 16. ABC. https://www.youtube.com/watch?v=53dumkxzHwA.

Hoar, Peter. 2021. *It's a Sin*, January 22–February 19. Channel 4. https://www.stan.com.au/watch/its-a-sin.

Lobl, Victor. 1983. *St Elsewhere*. S02,E09, Aids and Comfort. December 21. NBC. https://www.dailymotion.com/video/x7td531.

Nichols, Mike. 2003. *Angels in America*. December 7–14. HBO. https://binge.com.au/shows/show-angels-in-america!1515.

Pose. June 3, 2018 – June 6, 2021, FX. https://www.disneyplus.com/en-gb/series/pose/1ARtTsGv1oCS.

Queer as Folk. February 23, 1999 – February 22, 2000, Channel 4. https://www.stan.com.au/watch/queer-as-folk-1999.

Robe, Mike. 1988. *Go Toward the Light*, November 1. CBS. https://www.youtube.com/watch?v=0c23BIVWqdg.

Transparent. February 6, 2014 – September 27, 2019. Amazon Prime Video. https://www.amazon.com/Transparent-Season-1/dp/B089XSMKR4.

CHAPTER 4

Incorrigibility and Becoming-Child: Portrayals of People Living with HIV/AIDS in the Works of Cuban Writer Miguel Angel Fraga

Mirta Suquet

4.1 Introduction

The distinctive strategy of the Cuban government in managing the HIV/AIDS epidemic in the 1980s and 1990s had a significant influence on the development of a unique literary landscape within the wider narrative of HIV/AIDS in Latin America. Alongside the disease itself and the attending fear of death, issues arising from social segregation and implications of criminality due to compulsory isolation have become equally significant. The enforced quarantine policies in Cuba's 'AIDS sanatoriums' not only impacted public health but also led to significant human rights violations,

M. Suquet (✉)
Susquehanna University, Selinsgrove, PA, USA
e-mail: suquet@susqu.edu

A. Castillo Villanueva, A. Bollas (eds.), *HIV/AIDS in Memory, Culture and Society*, Palgrave Studies in Science and Popular Culture, https://doi.org/10.1007/978-3-031-59699-5_4

psychological distress, and feelings of isolation among the confined individuals.[1] Furthermore, Cuban literature on HIV/AIDS is inevitably shaped by institutional censorship and self-censorship among writers operating within a socialist political framework. This situation particularly impacts artists living with HIV/AIDS due to their precarious positions within the confines of the sanatoriums. Consequently, the Cuban literary corpus on HIV/AIDS remains relatively limited. These works faced delays in publication compared to their writing time, and some were ultimately published outside the country. Regrettably, certain works (including poems, short stories, and theatre pieces) produced within the sanatorium "Los Cocos" and debated in the sessions of the Literary Workshop "The Magic Mountain" never reached a wider readership within Cuba.[2]

This chapter focuses on the narratives authored by Miguel Angel Fraga during his time as a patient at the "Los Cocos" sanatorium from 1992 to 1996. These stories were compiled in the book *No dejes escapar la ira* [Don't Let Your Anger Escape], published in 2001, which remains the sole work of fiction published in Cuba dedicated entirely to the AIDS theme. The book delves into various perspectives, presenting viewpoints from a wide array of characters: patients, including both heterosexuals and homosexuals, *frikis*, chaperones, and families.

[1] In 1986, the inaugural sanatorium was established in Santiago de Las Vegas, located within the City of Havana. By 1991, these facilities had been set up across all provinces in the country, except for Las Tunas, Havana, and Isla de la Juventud. Their primary aim was to educate individuals on living with HIV, providing comprehensive medical and psychological care. From 1986 to 1989, stringent compliance with admission regulations was enforced, and visits or departures from the sanatorium were strictly regulated. During this period, the sanatorium was under military administration, with security guards. Residents were obliged to wear numbered pyjamas as outlined by the regulations. From 1989, the administration of the sanatorium transitioned to the Ministry of Public Health, leading to a relaxation of confinement measures, including the introduction of weekend passes and outings from the institution, either supervised or unsupervised. By 1994, the Ambulatory Care System was established, aimed at reintegrating HIV-positive individuals into society. A notable portion of these individuals returned to their homes, where they received comprehensive care from their family doctors. Alternatively, some chose to persist in residing within the sanatoriums (Aragonés López et al. 2007).

[2] Cuban literary workshops originated in the 1960s and became a nationally supported literary movement. These workshops, held regularly in community cultural centres and overseen by writers or art instructors, offered opportunities for young literature enthusiasts to engage in critical discussions about one another's literary works. The literary workshop "La Montaña Mágica" at the sanatorium commenced in 1992.

Additionally, I am interested in examining the intersection of these fictional stories with Fraga's non-fictional literary endeavours. Identified by the number 525 that marked his belongings and bedding in the sanatorium, Miguel Angel Fraga is also the author of two significant non-fiction books offering diverse perspectives on the initial 'AIDS sanatorium'. *En un rincón cerca del Cielo* [A Place Close to Heaven], published in 2008 (though based on material collected between 1994 and 1997), compiles twenty interviews of patients, family members, physicians, and support staff. Similarly, *Casa cercada. Diario de un sobreviviente* [Enclosed House: Diary of a Survivor], published in 2018, encompasses Fraga's diary written between 1992 and 1997. Both publications offer valuable insights into the various phases and transformations of the sanatorium, particularly focusing on the psychological traumas resulting from the confinement policy.

Fraga's books offer profound insights into how Cuba's official healthcare system persistently attempted to shape the identity of individuals living with HIV/AIDS. They were designated as irresponsible and morally deficient subjects during the early years of the sanatoriums, marked by stringent admission policies. His portrayal of the sanatorium experience highlights a pervasive sense of temporal stagnation, feelings of helplessness, and the psychological manipulation endured by patients, fostering a profound sense of constraint and control. These narratives reveal a prevailing paternalistic attitude within the sanatoriums, portraying individuals with HIV/AIDS as lacking autonomy and being infantilised, thereby challenging their individual rights within confinement. Fraga's stories also address the issue of the criminalisation of sexuality among HIV-positive individuals and the ongoing struggle for autonomy against institutional rules.

This chapter critically analyses the use of the 'incorrigible' category, drawing upon Michel Foucault's concept as depicted in Fraga's works to define individuals living with HIV in Cuban sanatoriums. Moreover, I aim to explore how the narrative portrayal of individuals living with HIV/AIDS reflects a negotiation process between 'sanatorium identities', deliberate acceptance of norms for survival, and methods employed to challenge disciplinary models. While patients in these institutions were often seen as infantilised, irresponsible, or treated as criminal subjects requiring constant correction, Fraga subverts this portrayal by presenting characters who consistently embody the 'incorrigible' label—rebels persistently defying authority. The emergence of the 'becoming-child' concept within the narrative serves as a political resistance, challenging enforced infantilisation and advocating for an experimental attitude that questions established norms. Fraga's writing serves as a means not only to resist structural and political violence but also to push back against the confinement in the sanatoriums and the mistreatment he endured. These narratives stand as compelling examples of resistance and serve as a testament to the memory of HIV/AIDS in Cuba, carrying implications for how we commemorate this history. Additionally, they carry substantial relevance in the contemporary context, demanding acknowledgement and reparations for the victims from the Cuban government.

4.2 The Cuban *Sidatorios and* 'Sanatorium Identities'

In 1986, the Cuban government established a nationwide programme to control the spread of HIV by channelling existing regulations protecting public health, such as Decree-Law 54, issued in April 1982. This decree empowered health authorities to implement extraordinary measures mandating compulsory quarantine to prevent the spread of disease and curtail activities posing health risks (Rodríguez Roch 1997, 182). Subsequently, these regulations facilitated the establishment of the *Santiago de Las Vegas Sanatorium* in Havana, known as "Los Cocos", specifically conceived for HIV-positive individuals where patients received medical and psychological care, as well as training in "Learning to Live with HIV", organised by psychologists from the sanatorium (Aragonés López et al., 2007).[3] Cuba replicated similar facilities across the country, opening thirteen centres and a correctional institution, where patients who breached the rules of the sanatoriums were sent—this primarily included those who attempted escape and were accused of potentially spreading the disease, despite the lack of effective evidence, as documented by Fraga and other artists such as filmmaker Iván Arocha (1992), as well as local and international

[3] The legality of isolation centres was ratified by Decree 139 on 4 February 1988. Article 123-C-1 stipulated that the Ministry of Public Health could carry out isolation of confirmed or suspected cases and other possible human reservoirs for the duration and at the location determined by the corresponding health authority (*Programa* 1997).

activists.[4] The sanatoriums offered essential services, including sustenance, accommodation, medication, social assistance, and intensive educational and preventive programmes.

The medico-legal apparatus in Cuba exacerbated the global notion of HIV/AIDS as an "epidemic of guilt" (Peterson 2000, 146), placing a stronger emphasis on confinement and control rather than public awareness campaigns. The country's policies not only confined HIV/AIDS patients but also stigmatised them, portraying them as socially perilous and disregarding their civic responsibilities. This approach not only resulted in human rights violations and the absence of confidentiality guarantees but also led to increased state expenditure, neglect of educational prevention strategies, and the fostering of a false sense of invulnerability to HIV among the population (Pérez-Stable 1992; Rodríguez Roch 1997).

The policies of social isolation for people living with HIV/AIDS in Cuba are a continuation of the biopolitical logics implemented by the Cuban Revolution since its triumph in 1959. These logics aim to control, channel, or remove from public space those individuals labelled as *antisociales*—including homosexuals, religious individuals, 'hippies', young peasants resisting collectivisation, and dissenting artists and intellectuals. The alleged reason for such measures is that these 'antisocials' promote beliefs and practices deemed subversive to official revolutionary values, closely linked to socialist morality and the ideal of the 'new man'—a productive worker, heterosexual, and fully dedicated to the demands of the socialist community (Guerra 2010, 268). A historical example illustrating this approach occurred from 1965 to 1968 with the establishment of the Military Units for Aid to Production (UMAP) facilities. During this period, over 30,000 and 40,000 young people were interned and subjected to forced labour, resulting in their imprisonment for periods of up to three years without formal charges (Guerra 2010, 268).

[4] The documentary *Al margen del margen* [Beyond the Margin] by Iván Arocha, filmed at "Los Cocos" in 1992, highlights, among various issues, the absence of a legal framework enabling patients to counter accusations of spreading the epidemic, an irony labelled by the filmmaker as "justicia revolucionaria" [revolutionary justice]. The Cuban Penal Code, in its Chapter V "Offenses against Public Health", addresses "Spread of Epidemics" in Article 187. Anyone who violates measures or provisions issued by health authorities or refuses to cooperate with them faces penalties ranging from imprisonment for three months to one year or a fine of 100 to 300 pesos or both. Furthermore, the law specifies that those who maliciously spread or facilitate the spread of a disease face imprisonment from three to eight years.

The emphasis on isolation in the context of AIDS was rooted in assumptions about the shameful origins of the disease and practices deemed deviant from the socialist model, in addition to systemic violence against homosexuality. However, the strictness of the quarantine on the basis of one's HIV-status varied over time, from mandatory internment between 1986 and 1989 to a more relative form of quarantine since the early 1990s. In 1991, a system was implemented that allowed individuals to leave the sanatorium accompanied by personnel affiliated with the institution.[5] This privilege was typically granted by the Comprehensive Evaluation and Orientation Commission (Comisión de Evaluación y Orientación Integral, CEOI), comprising members from nursing, social work, psychology, medicine, epidemiology, and psychiatry services. The commission's role was to assess the patient's *confiabilidad* [trustworthiness]. Consequently, those *confiables* were permitted to spend weekends at their homes, contingent upon having a "guarantor" or a reliable family member.[6]

Researchers emphasise Cuba's achievement in maintaining the lowest HIV infection rate and the highest level of AIDS treatment in the Caribbean region (Farmer 1999; Anderson 2009, 93; Scheper-Hughes 1993, 965; 2020). However, criticism arose due to the lengthy quarantine period, overshadowing this success. This contrast highlights the intricate balance between preserving public health and respecting the individual rights of citizens. As expressed by the Cuban writer Miguel Angel Fraga in the diary kept during his years at the Los Cocos sanatorium, he felt that "era uno de los elegidos para pagar el precio por la maldad del mundo. … Iba rumbo a un purgatorio para liberarme del ominoso pecado que cargaba sobre los hombros. A medio camino entre la realidad y el sueño, quizás iba a inmolarme como un mártir" (Fraga 2018, 19) [I was one of

[5] These chaperones, called "acompañantes" were individuals hired by the institution to monitor the patient during their outings from the sanatorium. At the end of the day, they were required to submit a detailed report about the places visited, people met, as well as any incidents that occurred. The relationships between the patients and the companions varied, but generally, they were hostile as they implied a violation of the patient's privacy (Fraga 2018, 88–91). The film *El acompañante* [*The Companion*] (2015) by Pavel Giroud focuses on the relationship between a sanatorium patient and his companion.

[6] The anthropologist Nancy Scheper-Hughes (1993, 966) explained that to ensure the *confiabilidad*, a commission "must be convinced that the resident understands and accepts that he or she is carrying potentially fatal, transmissible disease and that they have a moral obligation to see that no other person contracts it from them". However, this statement overlooks the subjectivity involved in the assessment by the commission members towards the patient, as well as the implicit biases that might influence such judgements.

those chosen to pay the price for the world's evil. ... Heading towards a purgatory to free myself from the ominous sin I carried on my shoulders. Halfway between reality and dream, perhaps I was going to sacrifice myself as a martyr]. This quote underscores the profound psychological impact of social stigma, portraying feelings of being victimised and morally judged. Ultimately, this leads Fraga to a sense of resignation and self-sacrifice. The notion of being singled out to shoulder society's perceived sins or wrongdoings implies taking on a sacrificial role, contemplating giving up personal well-being or even one's own life due to circumstances beyond one's control.

This self-perception can be linked to the realm of Cuban official discourse and practices, where a noticeable emphasis on prioritising collective well-being over individual welfare within the framework of socialist morality exists. This stance forms the core of the pedagogical and axiological structures that shape individuals in Cuba. The American doctor Ronald Bayer, an associate professor at Columbia University's School of Public Health, reported from his visit to "Los Cocos" sanatorium in 1988 that certain indoctrinated patients viewed their stay in the sanatorium as a revolutionary obligation, with one patient stating, "He was doing his part to defend the Cuban revolution", as quoted by Bayer (Zonana 1988).

Fraga seems to embody a heroic persona, fully aware of the guilt and societal stigma surrounding HIV/AIDS during that period. His mentioning of "sacrificing myself as a martyr" signifies a profound acceptance of the suffering he endures as a destiny imposed by external forces beyond individual control. The writer and professor Rafael E. Saumell described those interned in sanatoriums as "al mismo tiempo, pacientes y rehenes del estado" [simultaneously patients and hostages of the state], lacking the freedom to determine aspects of their life in the sanatorium. They were subjected to the control of those overseeing the internments, managing the healthcare system, and regulating the media, resulting in a loss of autonomy (Saumell 2011, 232–233). While initial strict security measures, such as tall walls, armed guards, and restricted family visits were relaxed post-1989, certain practices persisted within the sanatorium. These included obligatory cohabitation among patients, persistent exposure to illness and death among peers, comprehensive evaluations, restrictive measures, and a system of temporary leave permits from the institution. Many of the testimonies gathered in the volume *En un rincón cerca del cielo* (2008), edited by Fraga, emphasise the lasting psychological impacts experienced by patients due to these practices. The consequences of this isolation were profound, leading to enduring emotional distress and a persistent feeling of isolation, persisting even after their reintegration into society in 1996.[7]

Quoting a witness from *En un rincón*,

> Luego de haberme reinsertado socialmente, de haber regresado a los míos, nada es igual y en el fondo sigo sanatorizado. (…) En la calle, en mi trabajo, en mi casa, aún siento los estigmas que dejó el Sanatorio" (Fraga 2008, 200–201) [After reintegrating into society, returning to my familiar surroundings, nothing remains the same, and deep down, I still feel 'sanitarised'. (…). In the street, at work, at home, I continue to sense the lingering effects of the Sanatorium].

Removed from their social connections and community ties, individuals confined in Cuba's so-called AIDS sanatoriums or *sidatorios* reminiscent of those depicted in Thomas Mann's Davos Sanatorium, perceive themselves as entering an alternate spatial and temporal realm—a "state of limbo" experienced as "a life sentence for healthy people" (Leiner 2019, 116). In his diary, Fraga describes a sense of time stagnation, expressing that his actions are repetitive and lack a clear teleology or life purpose "[a]nclados, la vida transcurría sin prisas. … Conversábamos, esperábamos. No sé si esperábamos volver a conversar o morir" (2018, 68). [Anchored, life passed without haste. … We talked, we waited. I don't know if we hoped to talk again or to die.] On another occasion, referring ironically to the psychological manipulation to which the "patients" are subjected, leading to a nullification of their will, Fraga resorts to an element of fantasy that also alludes to the infantilisation of these subjects. Fraga expresses, "Nadie parece enfermo; tengo la impresión de que sirven una pócima en la comida para que perdamos la noción del tiempo y del orden" (Fraga 2018, 25–26). [No one appears unwell; I sense that they mix a potion into the food to disrupt our sense of time and order.] This subtle statement by Fraga highlights a crucial aspect concerning certain advantages of staying in the sanatorium during the profound economic crisis of the 1990s. In those times of crisis known as the "Special Period", having access to adequate food, just like the sanatorium patients, became a coveted privilege.

[7] Research conducted in the "Santiago de Las Vegas" Sanatorium in 1997 highlighted inadequate emotional support for HIV/AIDS patients, resulting in heightened anxiety, affecting learning and decision-making abilities, and emotional well-being. See Tamayo Baldoquin (2000).

Consequently, this situation caused the patients to somewhat overlook the government's human rights violations. Additionally, Marvin Leiner, in *Sexual Politics in Cuba*, sheds light on the prevailing ignorance about the difference between individuals diagnosed with AIDS and those who test HIV-positive but remain healthy, potentially never developing an AIDS-related illness. The enforced quarantine measures hardly address this lack of awareness of this distinction. The Cuban press often tagged sanatorium residents as 'AIDS Patients' (Leiner 2019, 132), leading both the general population and those diagnosed as HIV positive to erroneously believe that having the virus equates to imminent death. This perception somewhat contributed to justifying the confinement in sanatoriums, where patients could receive specialised care. For a person with HIV experiencing good health without symptoms, being hospitalised immediately classified them as a patient and, more significantly, as an unwell individual, impacting them psychologically. In his diary, Fraga expresses how, following his diagnosis, he felt devastated yet alive, still holding onto his plans for life. However, upon entering the sanatorium, he felt confined to a hospital bed, essentially labelled as sick just because he was a patient.

In the wake of escalating economic strain within the sanatoriums and a continuous surge in the number of occupants despite imposed control measures, it became evident that sustaining these facilities was not economically viable. Additionally, international pressure also impacted the internal regulations within the sanatoriums (de Gordon 2006).[8]

Consequently, compulsory quarantine regulations were loosened. Nevertheless, from 1997, individuals newly diagnosed with HIV were still required to undergo an eight-week educational program within a sanatorium. Upon completion of this program, patients were given the option to remain in the sanatorium. Concurrently, they were afforded the

[8] In 1988, the *Los Angeles Times* released one of the initial in-depth articles in the US media covering the Cuban HIV sanatorium system, detailing the visit of the first USA delegation to the facility. The article concluded by asserting that the implementation of a quarantine as a public health measure in response to HIV could only be described as "totalitarian" (Zonana 1988). Jonathan Mann, the first AIDS director at the World Health Organization, referred to the sanatoriums as "pretty prisons", according to the *New York Times* (McNeil Jr. 2012). Some Cuban doctors opposed the confinement of people living with HIV/AIDS in Cuba. D. Omar del Pozo Marrero wrote a letter in the 1980s to the Cuban Minister of Health, condemning the abuses within the sanatorium. He was imprisoned for over ten years. At the Sixth International AIDS Conference in San Francisco in 1990, Cuban doctors Dr Reinaldo Payá Sardiñas and Dr Antonio M. Gordon condemned Cuba's quarantine policies (de Gordon 2006).

opportunity to reintegrate into their communities, families, and workplaces while maintaining regular outpatient visits with their physicians. Ultimately, in 2006, the mandatory requirement of admission to a sanatorium was rescinded.

4.3 "Individuals to Be Corrected": Subjectivation and Self-Assertion in Fraga's Work

The works by Fraga analysed in this chapter delve into a representation that might be linked to 'the incorrigible' or 'the individual to be corrected', whose genealogy was traced by Michel Foucault in his lectures titled "The Abnormals", given at the Collège de France in 1975. This term was part of the trio of 'dangerous' individuals labelled as 'abnormals' in the nineteenth century and was examined in conjunction with the new dispositifs of bodily domestication. The emergence of the 'incorrigible' coincided with implementing disciplinary techniques observed in various institutions like the army, schools, and workshops during the seventeenth and eighteenth centuries. These new methods aimed to regulate bodies' behaviours, and capabilities, raising questions about those who resisted this normativity, no longer entirely subject to legal sovereignty.

This concept is instrumental in exploring its problematic reinterpretation in the late 1980s and mid-1990s, especially concerning individuals living with HIV in Cuban sanatoriums, as articulated in Fraga's literary works. Through his writings, Fraga illuminates the underlying pedagogical motives behind the establishment of sanatoriums and the broader concerns of the Cuban state in managing what is perceived as uncontrollable by an apprehensive authority.

This depiction reveals the pedagogical aim of the sanatorium and, more broadly, the Cuban state's concern with establishing numerous reeducation methods to manage what paranoid power views as uncontrollable. According to Foucault, the concept of the 'incorrigible' emerged during the eighteenth and nineteenth centuries, a period marked by the proliferation of medicalisation in private life and the reinforcement of contemporary subjectivation structures.

The distinguishing factor characterising the individual requiring correction is their incorrigibility. Paradoxically, this incorrigibility prompts a series of institutional interventions that surpass the usual methods of training and correction within family and conventional practices. It introduces a novel form of rectification or super-correction. Consequently, a dynamic interplay exists between incorrigibility and the potential for rectification encircling the individual needing correction (Foucault 2003, 58). As elucidated by Foucault, the individual targeted for correction differs from the monster in that it represents not an anomaly but rather an everyday occurrence (Foucault 2003, 58). The notion of incorrigible remains ambiguous and elusive: "being unable to provide any proof, we can never really demonstrate that an individual is incorrigible. He verges precisely on undecidability. We can offer no evidence or proof of incorrigibility" (Foucault 2003, 58). The expectation of recurring faults arises before they become evident. The very authority aiming to educate or reform the unmanageable ultimately determines their potential to be labelled as such.

Fraga's works shed light on the mechanisms of subjectification that impact the 'incorrigibles' within sanatoriums, a theme particularly explicit in *Casa cercada. Diario de un sobreviviente*. This text provides insights into the institutional frameworks and corrective measures imposed on patients, depicting them as irresponsible or morally deficient individuals often requiring continuous supervision and regulation. HIV infection is perceived as a moral failure, as Fraga notes in his diary, reflecting the shortcomings of Cuban training, disciplinary institutions, and mass organisations such as the Unión de Jóvenes Comunistas (Union of Young Communists) or the Comités de Defensa de la Revolución (Defense Committees of the Revolution). As these institutions failed in 'correcting' the individual, these individuals contract HIV. Once confined in the sanatorium, people living with HIV/AIDS, considered eternal incorrigibles, continue to be labelled as *no confiables* [untrustworthy], which perpetuates the repressive tendencies of the system. As Fraga ironically notes in his diary, illness was the reward for refusing to follow the aseptic and exemplary model of the new man (heterosexual, completely integrated into the tasks of the revolution). As a result, he had to remain "en el internado de los incorregibles" [in a boarding school made for incorrigibles] (Fraga 2018, 46).

Fraga's diary captures a poignant moment when he describes feeling debased, equating himself to the virus he carries: "Me sentí como un microbio" [I felt like a germ] (Fraga 2018, 44). This comparison underscores a duality within his identity—potentially perilous but also marginalised and dismissed. In a fragment of his diary, Fraga delves into a metaphorical exploration, likening his existence to that of a virus and ascribing characteristics of both aggression and self-defence against society's immune system: "Los poderosos linfocitos estatales nos mantienen cercados" [the powerful state lymphocytes keep us surrounded] (Fraga 2018, 127). This analogy appropriates the warlike metaphors often used to illustrate the replication of the virus within the body, hinting at a sense of purpose and moral complexity inherent in the condition—a notion cautioned by Susan Sontag in her renowned essay *AIDS and its Metaphors* (1989). The metaphorical warfare mirrors the oppressive power dynamics and control mechanisms observed within the institution, drawing an unsettling parallel between the writer's internal battles and the external environment's structured hierarchy.

Using the metaphor of the immune system, the writer draws a parallel with forms of governance that surpass the confines of the institution, projecting them into the realm of contemporary biopolitics. This approach visually encapsulates what Roberto Esposito (2012) has conceptualised as the "paradigm of immunization". According to the Italian philosopher, the paradigm of immunisation describes the tendency of modern societies to see themselves as organisms that must shield against external threats, with significant implications for social inclusion and exclusion. Esposito points out that this immune logic is evident in various social institutions and practices, where boundaries and barriers are established to safeguard the integrity of the social body. This includes the creation of national borders, the formulation of laws and regulations, and the implementation of security measures. The obsession with protection and defence may result in a loss of openness and the ability to coexist with differences.

In this passage, the 'Fraga-virus' traverses various offices and spaces within the sanatorium, undergoing assessment, medication, and control. Concurrently, in a retrospective manner, the Fraga-virus reflects on his journey to adulthood, the school and family bullying endured during the process of learning toxic masculinity, and the strategies devised to evade the immune surveillance system of the Cuban body/nation in the 1970s and 1980s as a gay individual, within the systemic violence of the Cuban Revolution against *conductas impropias* [improper conducts].[9] As the fragment concludes, the Fraga-virus, existing as a biological entity neither alive nor dead, and unable to be eradicated due to the absence of an effective vaccine, defiantly challenges the repressive mechanisms of the

[9] *Improper Conduct* is a documentary film from 1984, directed by Néstor Almendros and Orlando Jiménez Leal. The film conducts interviews with Cuban refugees to delve into the Cuban government's practice of imprisoning homosexuals compelling them into forced-labour camps called Military Units to Aid Production (UMAP) between 1965 and 1970.

'sanatorium-body' or the 'national-body' with its persistent presence and potential threat. In a state reminiscent of a zombie, he acknowledges his dependency on the sanatorium—similar to how viruses depend on cells—since, like viruses, he cannot sustain himself autonomously.

The mere perception of oneself being reduced to a virus that is unable to live outside the sanatorium evidently signifies a degradation of the human condition. In *Remnants of Auschwitz: The Witness and the Archive*, Giorgio Agamben refers to a quote by Primo Levi, explaining that "humanity and responsibility are something the deportee had to leave outside the camp's confines" (2000, 61). Levi described "liberation" as the moment when "we became men, that is, responsible beings" (quoted by Agamben 2000, 61). The absence of responsibility in such contexts is not only a legal deprivation, but it also signifies a fundamental moral erosion, highlighting the importance of human accountability and dignity. Linked to the suspension of responsibility, which denotes the ethical devaluation of an individual, philosopher Hannah Arendt explores how the prohibition of expressing emotions contributes to dehumanisation. In *On Violence* (1970), Arendt argues that certain systems of power dehumanise not when they inflict suffering, but when that suffering is unable to find expression through anger or violence. Arendt's cautionary note resonates, "not rage and violence, but their conspicuous absence is the clearest sign of dehumanization" (1970, 63). According to Arendt, rage is not merely a spontaneous reaction to suffering. It emerges when there is a belief that certain circumstances could be changed but remain unchanged, thus offending our sense of justice.

Considering Hannah Arendt's concepts, Fraga's chosen title for his collection of short stories stands out. *No dejes escapar la ira* hints at the importance of regulating emotions within disciplinary settings like the sanatorium. Hiding anger becomes a survival strategy for inmates dealing with authoritarian power. However, when Fraga brings this anger to light, he transforms it into an act of resistance rather than submission. This title originates in a story where a patient awaits the outcome of a "reliability assessment" conducted by the CEOI. In the story, a friend cautions the patient against displaying anger if the assessment yields unfavourable results, emphasising that an emotional outburst might lead to escalated confinement and corrective measures. He also advises caution when speaking. There is a strong tension in the story between what can be said and what the psychologist manages to "extract": "de lo que digas dependerán tus futuras salidas, no te dejes engatusar" (Fraga 2001, 51) [your future outings will depend on what you say, don't be deceived].

Fraga's diary (2018, 88) records that reliability assessments occurred every six months. Patients underwent a battery of tests, including intelligence and personality assessments, anxiety evaluations, self-appraisals, surveys about HIV/AIDS, and extensive interviews with psychologists, among other specifically designed assessments. Following this, the evaluation committee collated information from diverse sources, including feedback from companions tasked with monitoring the patient, and ultimately made a decision. All assessment techniques culminate in determining whether a patient is granted or denied the classification of 'confiable' [trustworthy]. The communication of test results frequently took over two weeks, leading to significant anxiety for the patients. Fraga describes it as a situation where the system assumes that testing HIV-positive equates to being mentally unstable and irresponsible until proven otherwise through a rigorous process. According to Marvin Leiner, the evaluation process can resemble an "Orwellian/Catch 22 nightmare", akin to being released from a mental hospital (Leiner 2019, 121). A positive assessment would grant temporary release from the sanatorium with a chaperone.

In several instances, the protagonists in the short stories of *No dejes escapar* contain their anger amid injustices or remarks from authority figures, meticulously controlling their emotions or responses during reliability tests. In his diary, Fraga notes that one of the primary motivations for his writing and gathering testimonials from other patients is to channel anger: "Escribo, escribo, escribo … Tal vez entre tanto destinador y destinatario, entre tantas bocas contando vidas y tantos oídos escuchando, se diga y se oiga la ira que llevamos dentro y que apenas dejamos escapar" [I write, I write, I write. … Perhaps amidst numerous senders and recipients, amid many voices recounting lives and many ears listening, the anger we harbour within will find expression and be heard—an emotion we seldom allow ourselves to let out] (Fraga 2018, 117).

Utilising a viral metaphor, it can be posited that the texts propagating anger function as subversive undercurrents, mirroring clandestine viral streams that infiltrate the established narratives surrounding the lives of individuals affected by HIV/AIDS in Cuba. Paradoxically, these viral texts have the power to reinstate a sense of humanity among those who testify to the injustices they have endured. In the book *Sida: Confesiones a un médico* [AIDS: Confessions to a Doctor], the director of Havana's sanatorium, Jorge Ángel Pérez, recounts life stories shared by his patients, the critique and visceral pulsation of anger captured by Fraga are often transformed into tears of regret and frustration due to the infection (or the prior 'incorrigibility' that led to the illness). Pérez, as stated in the book, decided to open the doors of the sanatorium to foreign visitors to "enseñar la verdad de Cuba ante las campañas internacionales de difamación" [to show the truth about Cuba amid international smear campaigns].[10] His book serves a similar purpose, emphasising the positive aspects of patient care at the sanatorium. However, by contrasting Fraga's works with Pérez's, a clear dissonance emerges concerning the differing perspectives from which these stories are narrated (from that of the patient or that of the "Patriarca", as Fraga refers to Pérez).

Included in *No dejes escapar*, the short story "*Mi Violencia es vivir*" [My Violence is to live] epitomises the figure of the 'incorrigible'. It narrates the tale of a young woman who injected herself with HIV-positive blood, an event that actually unfolded within marginalised urban tribes in 1990s Cuba, predominantly among the *frikis*.[11] Embracing a punk subculture in a society where Western rock music and the hippy lifestyle were seen as direct challenges to Communist ideology, the *frikis* represented a segment of non-conformist Cuban youth perceived as a threat to the values and principles of the Revolution. According to Patra Urairat (2021), while "the rest of the world saw the sanatoriums as prisons in disguise, the Frikis saw a unique opportunity (...), desperate to opt out of the collective. Faced with the choice of life under police brutality or in a state-supported clinic where food and drinks were free, many Frikis chose the latter". Some works discussing HIV self-injection in Cuba include the short film *Maldito*

[10] Fraga reveals how the sanatorium did indeed receive numerous international delegations. These delegations were escorted to the best housing areas and were only allowed to converse with those patients designated by the institution. In a repressive environment where each day the patient's status as "trustworthy" was at stake, it was expected that those offering testimony to the advantages of the Sanatorium turned out to be mouthpieces of power. Those who became spokespeople for the sanatorium were rewarded with improved living conditions or trips abroad as part of official delegations: "Pepona habló muy bien del Sanatorio. Por su lealtad le regalaron un sillón para que viera la televisión cómodamente" (Fraga 2018, 210). [Pepona spoke highly of the Sanatorium. Due to her loyalty, they gifted her a comfortable armchair to watch television]. On the contrary, those patients who wanted to testify before Human Rights representatives, as Fraga explains, were sentenced to prison (Fraga 2018, 87, 94).

[11] The exact number of Cubans who have self-injected HIV-positive blood is not officially documented in public statistics. However, estimates indicate that there are approximately 200 individuals across the country who have engaged in this practice (Prout 1999, 427).

sea tu nombre, Libertad (1993) [Cursed be your name, Freedom], directed by Vladimir Ceballos, which faced censorship in Cuba. Another notable production is the film *Socialism or Death*, by Swedish filmmaker Bengt Norborg, filmed clandestinely within Cuban sanatoriums in 1995 and broadcast in 1998. Furthermore, Cuban filmmaker Gerardo Chijona directed the feature film *Boleto al paraíso* [Ticket to Paradise], which was exhibited in Cuba in 2010.

The act of defiance, akin to numerous instances of resistance and intervention by subordinate individuals, is etched onto the body itself due to the lack of opportunities for negotiation in public and political discourse. This embodiment of protest transforms their bodies into symbols—wounds, blood, and virus—granting a voice to those regarded as subordinate. The illness seals a pact that reaffirms a dissident, self-destructive community, outside the boundaries of society or the nation, solidifying fraternal bonds that supersede the traditional familial connections, which are deemed ineffective or false. Paradoxically, the self-withdrawal from the revolutionary project—through future seclusion in the sanatoriums—allows these 'incorrigibles' to live on the margins, breaking the socialist identification between the individual and collectivity, and enclosing themselves within their own bodies.

The omniscient narrator of "Mi Violencia" presents a condensed biography of the main character, who comes from a humble background and a dysfunctional home. This background sets the stage for a series of missteps within the educational system that ultimately lead to drug consumption and self-injection with HIV-positive blood. In essence, the story could be situated in any contemporary urban context, except for the socialist society envisaged for Cuba. However, in the post-Soviet Cuba of the 1990s, the zones of socio-economic marginality resulting from the economic crisis become more starkly evident. As depicted in Fraga's story, that turn-of-the-century Cuba will possess more punitive technologies than effective educational ones: inevitably, the punitive cycle will ensnare the irredeemable ones at some point. According to Fraga, it is the system itself that, in attempting to re-educate and rigidly channel these individuals within pre-established models, produces them as marginal subjects. Consequently, their self-exclusion, secured by contracting HIV and confinement in the sanatorium, becomes a bodily inscription of the mechanisms of exclusion implemented by the authorities. The desire to find a community and a sense of belonging beyond the confines of the national community is, in itself, a political act. With the virus infection, the character in Fraga's story ultimately breaks free from the demands of socialist society, the presence of CDR guards, other mass organisations, and the police. Paradoxically, however, she faces the repressive rules of the sanatorium and the severe symptoms of the disease (Fraga 2001, 34–35).

Closely tied to the portrayal of patients in the sanatorium as 'incorrigible', the narratives reveal a paternalistic tactic that confines and shields Cubans living with HIV/AIDS: infantilisation. Foucault noted that psychiatry in the nineteenth century employed this strategy for intervention. Rather than demanding behaviour conform to a specific illness framework, the mere hint of infantilism was enough for psychiatry to intervene and classify the conduct as psychiatric (Foucault 2003: 304–305). The texts by Fraga depict a prevailing paternalistic attitude within the sanatorium that implies that individuals accept the authority of their "superiors" who provide them with protection and guidance. To access the perceived benefits of this paternalistic power, individuals are required to relinquish their claims to being treated as responsible adults worthy of respect (McGary 1992, 20). As a result, individuals are infantilised and become subjects in need of guidance, protection from the world and from their own actions, education, and continuous monitoring.

Similarly, all forms of paternalism necessitate that the intrusion or intervention be rationalised or justified by pointing to the good of the individual being intervened with, a certain incapacity or deficiency in the understanding of the person who is treated in a paternalistic manner, and the assessment made by the individual conducting the interference that they do indeed comprehend what is advantageous for this person (McGary 1992, 24).

As Howard McGary explains, advocates of paternalism historically argue for justified intervention in certain individuals' choices, even if the consequences primarily affect those individuals. Groups like children, women, individuals with disabilities, or neurodivergent individuals are often subjects of such intervention. Whether for utilitarian benefits, claiming that paternalism could maximise the societal usefulness of certain groups, or advocated for by human rights proponents emphasising the need to protect individuals from self-inflicted harm, paternalism implies a natural or socially constructed sense of imperfection and inferiority (McGary 1992, 22–23). At the level of the doctor-patient relationship, Nancy Mairs elucidates that "paternalism infects [medical professionals'] relations with all their patients—a word that does not share its root with 'passive' by accident—because [physicians'] apparent (and often real) power over life and death reduces us all to a childlike dependency on their superior knowledge" (Mairs 2002, 161). This dependency is reinforced by patients' compliance and submissiveness, contributing to the dominance of medical practitioners.

Fraga's diary and the testimonies compiled in *En un rincón*... reveal multiple instances of ableism and infantilisation practised by doctors, caregivers, chaperones, and leaders within the sanatorium. Fraga refers to the director of the sanatorium as the 'Patriarch' or 'The Omnipotent', denoting his authoritarian style. The patients consistently faced invasions of their privacy, dismissal, or belittlement of their wishes and opinions, and encountered various patronising discourses and practices. These ranged from the seemingly well-intentioned or encouraging to openly hostile, dehumanising, or more ambiguous forms. The loss of autonomy resulting from confinement policies consistently deprived individuals with HIV/AIDS of the ability to make significant decisions or assume responsibilities. This was particularly challenging given the medical and epidemiological uncertainty surrounding the emergence of the AIDS epidemic. In some passages of the diary, Fraga highlights the ethical quandary surrounding the forcible administration of treatment versus respecting patients' autonomy. For instance, there is a notable fragment where a nurse jokingly refers to patients as being physically and metaphorically constrained, perceived as the weakest link in the healthcare system and consequently disadvantaged (Fraga 2018, 73). As he sadly notes in his diary: "En este laboratorio somos marionetas al antojo de los que más y mejor mean" (2018, 210) [In this laboratory, we are mere puppets at the mercy of those who piss the most and best].

Additionally, the separation from their workplaces and the feeling of not actively contributing to the community, combined with constant reminders of the state's investment in their care and health, further reinforced the notion that people living with HIV/AIDS in Cuba were perceived as wards of the state, akin to children under its protection.

In Fraga's short story "Ay, Virgilio!" from *No dejes escaper la ira*, the condemnations of the patient's sexuality are portrayed as a ubiquitous and authoritarian voice that dominates the individual's consciousness, reducing them to an infantilised state and emphasising the degradation and suppression of their sexual autonomy: "no dejo de oír la voz que me escupe el sexo: desnúdate hombre, muchacho, niño: muestra tus inhibiciones, tu sexo minúsculo, insignificante. Ahora eres un escolar, apenas un adolescente. En lo adelante te condeno al onanismo" (Fraga 2001, 131)

[I cannot stop hearing the voice that spits on my sex: undress, man, boy, child: show your inhibitions, your tiny, insignificant sex. Now you are a schoolboy, barely a teenager. From now on, I condemn you to masturbation].

According to Scheper-Hughes (1993, 963), each patient was obligated to adhere to "the three commandments of the sanatorium": engaging in unprotected sex with an unknowing, uninfected individual was deemed murder; having unsafe but consensual sex with an uninfected partner was considered criminal; and engaging in unprotected sex with another infected partner was viewed as mutual suicide. These 'commandments' underscore the prevailing moral code that governed the sanatorium, categorising diverse sexual behaviours on moral grounds. However, one might question the relevance of employing such stringent legal and moral terms within the context of illness, along with the potential subjectivity and inflexibility of these rules in practical application.

The criminalisation of sexuality is discernible in some of Fraga's short stories from *No dejes escapar*, where characters unintentionally breach some of the 'three commandments' of the sanatorium, risking being adjudged guilty by the courts for spreading the disease and consequently facing imprisonment. These narratives illuminate the moral nuances embedded in sexuality, decisions regarding partners, and romantic sentiments. Ultimately, the stories appeal to an individual's capacity to make informed and consensual choices, even when these decisions contradict state regulations.

In "El otro Miguel", Fraga highlights the shortcomings of the official policy addressing the HIV epidemic, exposing a system tainted by legal interventions that overlook the intricacies of intersubjective relationships and the complex interplay of desire, sex, love, and disease. The central character faces accusations of unintentionally transmitting the disease to their partner during an authorised leave from the institution. While the infection occurs accidentally, this tragic turn ultimately forges the desired union for both, enabling them to coexist in the sanatorium and confront the challenges posed by the disease. As articulated in the text, the partner of the person living with HIV/AIDS accepts her diagnosis, given that for her, enduring the absence of her husband, the sporadic visitation regime imposed by quarantine, and other impediments become more unbearable than the fear of falling ill: "[L]a felicidad es estar junto a Miguel, ser su otra persona, el otro ser de su agonía" (2001, 76) ["[H]appiness lies in being with Miguel, being his other self, the alternate entity in his suffering"]. The plot takes an absurd turn when the partner assumes Miguel's place in the sanatorium, as Miguel is transferred to jail, accused of intentionally spreading HIV. Due to the unsanitary conditions in jail, the disease's symptoms intensify: "Fue trasladado al hospital días antes de su muerte y su muerte añadió un número más a los números de una computadora" (2001, 77). [He was transferred to the hospital days before his death, and his death added one more number to the numbers in a computer]. The focus on statistics highlights the dehumanisation of the individual within a system geared towards epidemiological control.

The short story "Si la suerte me roza la cara" [If Luck Grazes my Face] tackles the controversial issue of parenthood among individuals infected with HIV, which was a hotly debated topic within Cuban health policies. During the period of strict isolation in sanatoriums, doctors often recommended terminating pregnancies, leading most pregnant women to yield to pressure from health authorities.[12] Between 1986 and 2002, 868 women were reported to be HIV/AIDS positive, of which only 92 decided to pursue their pregnancies (González Núñez et al. 2004). More than half of the pregnancies were reported after 1997, when the reintegration of people living with HIV/AIDS into society was regularised ("El sida y el dilema de maternidad", 2002). The main character of "Si la suerte ...", who is HIV-positive, holds on to the probabilities provided by doctors that the child his wife is expecting might be born healthy and advocates for his right to become a father. This short story unfolds as a narrative dialogue, where the patient challenges the opinions of an authoritative figure (such as a doctor or a psychologist), highlighting the ongoing clash of representations within these texts. The character is depicted as existing within a constant struggle between what is expected of him (reflected in the voices permeating the narrative) and his personal deliberations, always feeling the need to explain and justify himself.

The discussed texts delve into the interplay between the micro-politics of personal experiences and the macro-politics of state control. These narratives underscore the portrayal of individuals living with HIV/AIDS as

[12] See "El sida y el dilema de maternidad" (https://ipsnoticias.net/2002/11/salud-cuba-el-sida-y-el-dilema-de-maternidad/). Among the various testimonies compiled by Fraga in *En un rincón*, there is the account of Nivia, an HIV-positive mother who underwent an abortion at six and a half months pregnant in 1988. Subsequently, when she became pregnant again, she faced the punishment of being unable to leave the institution. Afterward, she was sentenced to one year in prison. However, her daughter was born healthy (Fraga 2008, 227–231).

individuals striving to assert autonomy within the oppressive confines of the sanatorium. These individuals resist succumbing to the biopolitical logics enforced through a system of constraints and regulatory measures on bodies with HIV/AIDS, aimed at curtailing flows, relationships, and, ultimately, transmissions. Nevertheless, an excess flow escapes control. In this context, the characters affirm the power of emotions and desires, thus embodying an incorrigible spirit that seeks to resist domestication.

4.4 Incorrigibility and Becoming-Child: Modes of Resistance Against Power

In the following pages, I explore the concept of 'incorrigibility' through the lens of the creative and resistant capacity demonstrated by the characters in Fraga's works. Fraga illustrates how patients exhibit resourcefulness in navigating strict norms, persistently seeking moments of freedom, even when these are precarious or fleeting, and challenging the quarantine regimen and institutional mechanisms of control and correction.

Through various short stories, the writer portrays individuals who find ways of reinventing themselves behind the walls of the sanatorium and lead a bearable and, to a certain extent, happy life. In such cases, this involves embracing a challenging vitality and optimism that supersedes the logic of the sanatorium as a hospital for incurable or dying patients. This thematic exploration is exemplified in the text "Gunilla", inspired by Guillermo Ginestá, a drag queen celebrated for performances within the sanatorium. The narrative unfolds in the form of an interview, brimming with liveliness, and a palpable sense of excitement as Gunilla prepares for the show. Gunilla, the 'diva', elucidates to the narrator that within the sanatorium, particularly among the homosexual community cohabiting in the same area, she could freely explore her artistic inclinations. This would have been challenging or even perilous for Ginestá to do outside the sanatorium, given the prevalent homophobia and transphobia in society.[13] Likewise, Fraga's diary is replete with references to acts of rebellion, pro-

[13] This show and many other initiatives were driven by the patients themselves. "Nosotros mismos inventamos los espacios y las formas para hacer más llevadera nuestra vida" (Fraga 2018, 79) [We invented spaces and ways to make our lives more bearable], Fraga says in his diary, narrating how they organized costume parties, set up a disco in an abandoned space, and created the drag queen show by crafting their own dresses from scraps and curtains, among numerous other stagings of a startling effeminate behaviour they didn't aim to conceal.

test, and defiance carried out by the sanatorium patients. Throughout, there are accounts of patients frequently fleeing the sanatorium to visit their relatives, well aware of the severe repercussions that will ensue. Some manage to procure drugs for recreational use (Fraga 2018, 65), while others cleverly outmanoeuvre the guards by using ingenious methods to smuggle alcoholic beverages into the sanatorium (67). In his attempt to document the unique experiences of his peers, Fraga provides accounts of more radical forms of opposition, such as the alienation experienced by some patients, the suicide attempts of others, or the intentional transmission of the virus to enter the sanatorium, including the self-injection of HIV by the *frikis*. The embodiment of protest through physical inscriptions becomes notably significant when "Fito, el irreverente" [Fito, the irreverent] tattoos a barbed wire bracelet onto his hands in protest and defiance: "cuando los extranjeros nos visiten en los Cocos, no tendrán necesidad de preguntar nada. Les enseño mis muñecas y que saquen ellos sus propias conclusions" [When foreigners visit us at Los Cocos, they won't need to ask anything. I show them my wrists and let them draw their own conclusions] (2018, 79).

Another form of resistance to power, opposing the "infantilisation" of HIV patients within the constructed sanatorium-induced identities, recalls Deleuze and Guattari's concept of "becoming-child" and its potential political significance. Daan Keij, following Guattari's insights, elucidates that "infantilization is mainly characterized by homogenization (…) [T]he link between infantilization and homogenization seems to consist of the breakdown of critical maturity (infantilization) which is then replaced with standardized identities and modes of living (homogenization)" (Keij 2022). While "infantilization produces a mass of homogenized subjectivities" (Keij 2022), "becoming-child", in contrast, signifies adopting an experimental attitude that incites actions in entirely unforeseen ways, challenging prevailing norms (Keij 2022). Walter Kohan explains that "becoming-child" functions as a war machine against the state and adult institutions. As a non-sequential progression, it encapsulates a space of resistance, a departure from established norms, a latent potential, a source of creativity, and other ways of affecting and being affected by the world (Kohan 2012, 173).

In the context of the sanatorium, "becoming-child" signifies a refusal to succumb to the process that ensures the infantilisation of patients or that they behave in conformity with the expected model of a responsibility imposed by authority figures. While technologies of education, surveillance, psychological interventions, and punishment adhere to a teleology of 'growing up', wherein the patient-child undergoes a process of maturation segmented in stages and consisting in preparing to assume responsible adulthood, "becoming-child" emerges as something contrary and resistant to the normative identity of an "adult" in society. It is a line of flight, a trajectory of escape deterritorialising the father's law (Kennedy, 2013).

The short story "Nalgas al fondo" [Bottoms Up], featured in *No dejes escapar*, centres on portraying the liberating potency of a character who, in my view, embodies certain aspects of Deleuze's concept of "becoming-child". The narrative recounts several episodes featuring this singular character: the celebration he organised to inform his friends about his virus status, his jovial, mischievous, and carefree nature that leads him to mock death, his own and that of his peers, and, particularly, how he outwitted the supervisors accompanying him on his excursions from the sanatorium. Intent on maintaining his sexual activity responsibly despite strict prohibitions, he employs shrewd strategies that subtly challenge authority. For instance, he administers sleeping pills to the chaperone in the café and escapes through the room windows while the chaperone is asleep. He even resorts to bribing the chaperone with gifts, among other tactics. He embodies a rebellious spirit, seeking alternative routes to seek satisfaction and disrupt the established norms within the boundaries of the sanatorium.

After his death from complications related to AIDS, the family 'adultified' the main character's image: "la imagen en el féretro, peinado como nunca lo hizo, mostrando una cara que no era la suya. Una expresión ridícula. ... Todos tratan de distorsionar tu verdadera imagen, mostrarte a su conveniencia" [the image in the coffin, his hair styled in a way he never did, displaying an unrecognizable face. A ludicrous expression. Everyone tries to distort your true image, to display you to their convenience] (2001, 106). However, neither the narrator nor the rest of the friends will remember him as "corrected", but rather as an intense character who challenged authority (2001, 106).

Through the dual portrayal of both the authentic and post-mortem corrected images in his text, Fraga encapsulates the relentless resistance carried out by his characters to prevent the erasure of their identities. In a poignant excerpt from his diary, Fraga highlights the Cuban media's portrayal of HIV/AIDS patients living in sanatoriums, expressing how their faces have been obliterated from representation. Confronting the official prevention campaign's slogan, "El sida no tiene cara" [AIDS has no face],

Fraga reflects: “Pienso que sí tiene cara: la mía, la de Muñequero, la de Enfermero … caras muy distintas que podrían contar sus experiencias y llegar a más gente. En cambio, nos encierran, nos borran el rostro. Visto así, en efecto, *el sida no tiene cara*” [I believe it does have a face: mine, Muñequero’s, Enfermero’s … distinct faces capable of narrating their experiences and connecting with more people. Instead, they confine us, efface our identities. In this context, indeed, AIDS seems faceless] (55).

The work of Miguel Angel Fraga on HIV/AIDS counters this erasure by depicting the characters’ resilience, rebellious acts, and their capacity to carve out liveable existences within restrictive settings. The stubborn incorrigibility and process of “becoming-child” among specific characters emerge as strategies of resistance against the enforced infantilisation of HIV/AIDS patients within the sanatorium’s controlling structures. These challenges and resistances encountered by the characters represent direct confrontations against the predetermined “responsible” identities imposed by governing authorities.

In conclusion, Miguel Angel Fraga’s narratives, particularly those originating from his experiences within the Los Cocos sanatorium, hold significant value in the context of HIV/AIDS representation in Cuba. Fraga’s literary contributions not only serve as an exploration of the individual’s struggle for autonomy within the oppressive environment of the sanatorium but also function as powerful resistance narratives against governmental control and biopolitical logics. The delayed publication and limited circulation of Fraga’s works within Cuba underscore the impact of institutional censorship on the depiction of the epidemic.

Beyond the literary realm, Fraga’s narratives contribute to the collective memory of HIV/AIDS, serving as a testament to the experiences of those confined in the sanatoriums and shedding light on the human rights violations and psychological distress endured. The significance of Fraga’s work extends beyond its initial creation, influencing the present-day discourse on Cuba and HIV. It prompts reflection on the current status of HIV/AIDS in Cuba, as well as any recognition or acknowledgement given to the victims of the sanatoriums. In doing so, Fraga’s narratives underscore the enduring role of literature in shaping perspectives, challenging historical narratives, and creating new meanings surrounding HIV/AIDS, ensuring that the memory of these experiences remains relevant and impactful for future generations.

References

Agamben, Giorgio. 2000. *Remnants of Auschwitz: The Witness and the Archive*, eBook. New York: Zone Books.

Almendros, Néstor, and Orlando Jiménez Leal, directors. 1984. *Conducta Impropia*. Les Films du Losange and Antenne 2. DVD Video.

Anderson, Tim. 2009. HIV/AIDS in Cuba: A Rights-Based Analysis. *Health and Human Rights* 11 (1): 93–104.

Aragonés López, Carlos, Campos Díaz, Jorge Raúl, et al. 2007. Grupos de Prevención del SIDA (GPSIDA): 15 años de trabajo sostenido en la prevención del VIH/sida. *Revista Cubana de Medicina Tropical* 59 (3) http://scielo.sld.cu/scielo.php?script=sci_arttext&pid=S0375-07602007000300014. Accessed 20 Dec 2023.

Arendt, Hannah. 1970. *On Violence*. New York: Harcourt Brace Jovanovich.

Arocha, Iván, director. 1992. *Al margen del margen* [Film]. https://www.cubaencuentro.com/multimedia/videos/sida-en-cuba-al-margen-del-margen. Accessed 20 Dec 2023

Ceballos, Vladimir, director. 1993. *Maldito sea tu nombre, Libertad*. VHS.

Chijona, Gerardo, director. 2010. *Boleto al paraíso*. Kimbara Cine Cubano, DVD Video.

de Gordon, Antonio M. 2006. VIH-SIDA en Cuba: Actualización 2006. https://healtheducationresources.unesco.org/sites/default/files/resources/2006_VIH_SIDA_en_Cuba_Actualizacion.pdf. Accessed 20 Dec 2023

Esposito, Roberto. 2012. Community, Immunity, Biopolitics. *Política común*. Vol 3, Michigan: University of Michigan Library. https://quod.lib.umich.edu/p/pc/12322227.0003.001?view=text;rgn=main. Accessed 20 Dec 2023.

Farmer, P. 1999. *Infections and Inequalities: The Modern Plagues*. Berkeley: University of California Press.

Foucault, Michel. 2003. *Abnormal. Lectures at the Collège de France 1974-1975*. London: Verso.

Fraga, Miguel Ángel. 2001. *No dejes escapar la ira*. La Habana: Letras Cubanas.

———. 2008. *En un rincón cerca del cielo. Entrevistas y testimonios sobre el SIDA en Cuba*. Valencia: Aduana Vieja.

———. 2018. *Casa cercada. Diario de un sobreviviente*. Madrid: Ediciones La Palma.

Giroud, Pavel, director. 2015. *El acompañante*. Habanero International Sales. DVD Video.

González Núñez, Díaz Jidy, et al. 2004. Terapia antirretroviral en gestantes seropositivas al VIH/SIDA en Cuba. *Revista Cubana de Medicina Tropical* 56 (1). http://scielo.sld.cu/scielo.php?script=sci_arttext&pid=S0375-07602004000100013. Accessed 20 Dec 2023

Guerra, Lillian. 2010. Gender Policing, Homosexuality and the New Patriarchy of the Cuban Revolution, 1965-70. *Social History* 35 (3): 268–289.

Inter Press Service. Periodismo y Comunicación para el cambio global. 2002. Salud, Cuba: El sida y el dilema de maternidad, November 27. https://ipsnoticias.net/2002/11/salud-cuba-el-sida-y-el-dilema-de-maternidad/. Accessed 20 Dec 2023

Keij, Daan. 2022. The Risks of a Recurring Childhood: Deleuze and Guattari on Becoming-Child and Infantilization. *Educational Philosophy and Theory.* https://doi.org/10.1080/00131857.2022.2128759. https://www.tandfonline.com/doi/full/10.1080/00131857.2022.2128759?scroll=top&needAccess=true. Accessed 20 Dec 2023.

Kennedy, David. 2013. Becoming Child, Becoming Other: Childhood as Signifier. In *Childhood in the English Renaissance*, ed. Anja Muller, 145–153. Trier: Wissenschaftlicher Verlag Trier.

Kohan, Walter Omar. 2012. Childhood, Education, and Philosophy: Notes on Deterritorialisation. In *Philosophy for Children in Transition: Problems and Prospects*, 170–189. Chichester, UK: Wiley-Blackwell.

Leiner, Marvin. 2019. *Sexual Politics in Cuba: Machismo, Homosexuality, and AIDS.* New York: Routledge.

Mairs, Nancy. 2002. Sex and Death and the Crippled Body: A Meditation. In *Disability Studies: Enabling the Humanities*, ed. Sharon L. Snyder, Brenda Jo Bruggemann, and Rosemarie Garland-Thomson, 156–170. New York: Modern Language Association.

McGary. 1992. *Between Slavery and Freedom: Philosophy and American Slavery.* Bloomington: Indiana University Press.

McNeil Jr., Donald G. 2012. Cuba's Fortresses Against a Viral Foe. *The New York Times.* May 7. https://www.nytimes.com/2012/05/08/health/cubas-aids-sanitariums-fortresses-against-a-viral-foe.html. Accessed 20 Dec 2023

Norborg, Bengt, director. 1998. *Socialism or Death.* Sveriges Television. VHS Video.

Pérez, Jorge Ángel. 2008. *Sida: Confesiones a un médico.* Ciudad de La Habana: Casa Editora Abril.

Pérez-Stable, Eliseo J. 1992. La epidemia del SIDA en Cuba. *Revista Latinoamericana de Psicología* 24 (1–2): 71–84.

Peterson, Christopher. 2000. Resenting Aids: paranoia, punishment, performativity. *Qui Parle* 12 (1): 145–176.

Programa Nacional de Control y Prevención del VIH/SIDA. 1997. Ministerio De Salud Pública. https://instituciones.sld.cu/ipk/files/2012/07/sida.pdf. Accessed 20 Dec 2023.

Prout, Ryan. 1999. Jail-House Rock: Cuba, AIDS, and the Incorporation of Dissent in Bengt Norborg's Socialism or Death. *Bulletin of Latin American Research* 18 (4): 423–436.

Rodríguez Roch, Liana. 1997. El sida en Cuba. *Papers: Revista de Sociologia* 52: 177–186.

Saumell, Rafael E. 2011. Finca Los Cocos: El primer sanatorio para enfermos de SIDA en Cuba. In *Cuba: Arte y Literatura en el exilio*, ed. Grece Piney and James J. Pancrazio, 227–237. Valencia: Legua Editorial.

Scheper-Hughes, Nancy. 1993. AIDS, Public Health, and Human Rights in Cuba. *The Lancet*, October 16, 965–967.

———. 2020. Cuba HIV/AIDS: Epidemics and Containment. *Berkeley News*, June 22. https://news.berkeley.edu/2020/06/22/cuba-hiv-aids-epidemic-epidemics-and-containment. Accessed 20 Dec 2023.

Tamayo Baldoquin, María M. 2000. Qué espera de la enfermera con respecto al tratamiento emocional el paciente con Virus de Inmunodeficiencia Humana. *Revista Cubana de Enfermería* 16 (1): 25–33.

Urairat, Patra. 2021. Los Frikis: The Cubans Who Infected Themselves with HIV. *The Iris*, April 4. https://www.theirisnyc.com/post/los-frikis-the-cubans-who-infected-themselves-with-hiv. Accessed 20 Dec 2023.

Zonana, VF. 1988. Cuba's AIDS Quarantine Center Called 'Frightening.' *The Los Angeles Times*, November 4. https://www.latimes.com/archives/la-xpm-1988-11-04-mn-1196-story.html. Accessed 20 Dec 2023.

CHAPTER 5

Remembering 'Risky' Sex: Viral Hauntology and Post-crisis Cruising Discourses

David O'Mullane

5.1 Remembering 'Risky' Sex: Viral Hauntology and Post-crisis Cruising Discourses

In *Thinking Sex*, Rubin (1984) describes how Western cultures judged sexual acts within a moral hierarchy of good and bad behaviours. In this framework, monogamous sex between married heterosexuals was the height of respectability, whereas queer promiscuity was intuitively understood as corrupting and immoral. Rigidly policing the boundaries of "this erotic DMZ" ensured "something unspeakable [did not] skitter across" (282) to pollute a heteronormative public realm. This manner of sexual moralising—what Rubin terms "the domino theory of sexual peril" (282)—is evident in early responses to the AIDS pandemic as a *contrapasso* link was established between the promiscuity of the 1970s sexual revolution and the emergence of the disease in the 1980s. Panic and fear were undoubtedly the dominant affective states of the early years of the AIDS

D. O'Mullane (✉)
Dublin City University, Dublin, Ireland
e-mail: david.omullane2@mail.dcu.ie

A. Castillo Villanueva, A. Bollas (eds.), *HIV/AIDS in Memory, Culture and Society*, Palgrave Studies in Science and Popular Culture, https://doi.org/10.1007/978-3-031-59699-5_5

pandemic (Watney 1987; Crimp 2002). However, in *Positive Images* (2018), Kagan explores how the anxieties that abounded in the crisis years are not a thing of the past; they persist as a ghostly "unresolved presence" (7) in the cultures of the Global North. The 'post-crisis' period is defined by advances in the treatment and prevention of HIV, but the "whore cultures of liberation" (219) still haunt ideas about queer sex in the present.[1]

Hauntology is used by Derrida (1994) to explain the agency of the past in the present: how previous historical events and political ideas appear as ghostly revenants in contemporary sociopolitical issues and debates. Møller and Ledin (2020) adapt the concept to their analysis of contemporary HIV prevention strategies using viral hauntology to describe how older, morality-driven perspectives on sex recur in discourses on queer sexual behaviours today. However, the hauntological dimensions of the AIDS pandemic—the feelings of loss and the affective echoes of trauma—also inform anti-homonormative, queer and sex-positive perspectives on dissident sex. Viral hauntology influences how, in the post-crisis era, "gay communities imagine gay sexual sociability to be virtuous, sustainable, transgressive" (148) and political. By examining post-crisis cultural artefacts that represent and memorialise cruising cultures, this chapter adopts a hauntological approach to explore how recollections of the sexual past imbue contemporary queer promiscuity with contradictory political and moral significations.[2]

Haunting is a particularly apt metaphor for understanding the cultural impact of HIV/AIDS because, as Wendy Brown (2001) explains, ghosts can be manipulated; they can "be conjured and exorcised" (151) in ways that shape understandings of the past and present. Muñoz touches on the queer implications of this in *Cruising Utopia* (2009), pointing out how the abject "spectre of public sex [...] performs the illicit" (46) for

[1] Kagan's (2018) use of the term 'post-crisis' refers to the period after the introduction of antiretroviral drugs in 1996. However, its use does not imply the HIV/AIDS pandemic is 'over' in any real sense. Instead, it describes how, in the Global North, understandings of HIV/AIDS have shifted from "a state of crisis to one of chronicity" (15).

[2] Cruising is the subcultural practice of seeking out and identifying potential sexual partners in public space. The practice developed as a tactical response to the policing of homosexuality as people had to develop visual or verbal codes that privately signalled their sexuality. Although commonly referred to as 'public sex', cruising cultures also encompass semi-public, sex on-premises type environments such as bathhouses, saunas, sex theatres and sex clubs. From a contemporary standpoint, cruising has evolved into the digital realm with the location-based hook-up app Grindr allowing queer people to cruise anywhere they have phone service.

homonormative politics, allowing clear demarcations to be made between progressive good gay behaviours and regressive bad ones.[3] Likewise, Kagan's (2018) recent examination of contemporary media representations of 'risky' sexual practices, such as barebacking and chemsex, demonstrates how the restless spectre of the "polluting, promiscuous hedonist faggot" (21) stands as a potent warning against abandoning oneself to narcissistic pleasure. By examining John Walter's 2015 exhibition *Alien Sex Club*, this chapter details that—despite advances in the treatment and prevention of HIV—promiscuity is still cast as a recidivist, risk-laden behaviour.

5.2 Panic in the Alien Sex Club

John Walter was compelled to create *Alien Sex Club* as a response to a reported rise in HIV diagnoses among men who have sex with men (MSM) in the UK in 2012 (Aghaizu et al. 2013).[4] Walter collaborated with HIV specialist Dr Alison Rodger on his exhibition, which was funded, in part, by the Wellcome Trust and the Terrence Higgins Trust.[5] A vocal proponent of a maximalist aesthetic, Walter designed a cacophonous and colourful cruise maze dense with paintings, video pieces and sculptures to explore his post-crisis perspective on sexual health and gay sex. By recontextualising biomedical discourses in a ludic format, Walter (2016) believed he could educate audiences on the issue of HIV and "help reduce rates of transmission" (26). However, a close reading of some of the paintings in *Alien Sex Club* reveals how Walter sought to reinvigorate an affective state of panic concerning cruising and HIV transmission. In *Sex Clubs in Perspective* (2015), Walter incorporated viral capsids directly into the schematic of a sex club. The title implies that the viewer is witnessing the hid-

[3] Abjection, as Julia Kristeva (1982) and Barbara Creed (1993) have highlighted, is a process based on a confronting encounter with otherness that defines and affirms the boundaries and norms of the dominant order.

[4] The report in question showed men who had sex with men (MSM) "accounted for 3250 (51%) of new diagnoses in 2012, the highest ever reported" (Aghaizu et al. 2013, p. 9). However, it is important to note that the authors stressed that these increases were "difficult to interpret in isolation" and could be attributed to increased HIV testing among gay men in addition to "ongoing high rates of transmission" (9). Despite this, Walter utilised the study to establish and explore a causal link between cruising and HIV transmission.

[5] Dr Rodger was the lead author of the PARTNER1 and PARTNER2 studies which unambiguously demonstrated that people on effective HIV antiretroviral treatment cannot transmit the HIV (Rodger et al. 2016, 2018).

den 'truth' of these spaces as sites of viral transmission. In doing so, Walter invoked the longstanding "spatial metaphor of the cesspool" (Kagan 2018, 37), which originated in cholera outbreaks in the nineteenth century. As Kagan (2018) notes, sexual spaces like tearooms and bathhouses were metaphorically bound to the cesspool in the crisis years because it was believed they fostered "perverse sexualities and transmissible disease" (37). Walter's painting *Icarus in Vauxhall* (2015) reanimated this spatial metaphor in its depiction of the eponymous winged figure, mouth agape in horror, plunging to his death. According to *The Dictionary of Subjects and Symbols in Art*, Icarus's sorry flight was regularly deployed by Renaissance moralists as an allegory on the virtues of temperance (Hall 2018, 159). Icarus's descent is superimposed over another sex club schematic, a clear statement that these spaces are the home of fallen figures.

Walter (2016) assumed a causal link existed between HIV transmission and cruising spaces because they facilitated a risky "culture of meeting strangers for sex" (25). However, Frank (2019), in her in-depth review of the literature on collective sex venues, stresses that although studies have often conceptualised them as risk-laden spaces, close examination reveals the myriad ways in which participants care for themselves and others through the implementation of safe sex and "risk reduction practices" (7). For example, studies have shown that people who visit cruising spaces are tested for HIV at vastly higher rates than the general population (Daskalakis et al. 2009; Gama et al. 2017). Although Walter (2016) claimed that the goal was to "show the contemporary reality of HIV" (2), he was drawn to older sex panic discourses as evidenced by his repeated use of the familiar bogeymen of HIV transmission: the barebacker, the bug chaser and the gift giver.[6]

Octavio Gonzalez (2019) explains that these HIV folk devils operate as "panic icons" for a seronegative audience. They "discipline the uninfected, to encourage them to continue protecting themselves from HIV" (51).[7] Much like Walter visually tied the cruiser to ideas of disease, addiction and death, seropositive individuals featured in *Alien Sex Club* as monstrous *panic icons* of viral transmission. For example, the painting *This is the*

[6] A barebacker is someone who has sex "without a condom," a bug chaser is an "HIV negative person looking to get infected with HIV," while a gift giver is an "HIV positive person looking to infect someone who is not infected with the virus" (Walter 2016, 22).

[7] In the context of HIV, seronegativity means a person does not have circulating antibodies for the HIV virus.

Initiation of the Bug Chaser depicted a man being branded with the symbol denoting his status as a bug chaser.[8] The seropositive individual, the gift giver, was dehumanised into a grotesque hybrid between man and virus, his head an HIV capsid replete with glycoprotein protuberances. Walter (2016) readily admitted he was aware of "the controversial or disputed nature" of bug chasing and gift giving, but felt they were important to use as "[he] found the language and mythology of seroconversion rich in imagery and ideas" (197). Walter's reinvestment in *abjectifying* scare tactics arguably stemmed from his belief that fear was a useful way of modifying behaviours and reducing viral transmission. His overarching goal was to generate an *affective* state of crisis. By anxiously assessing their exposure to risk, a seronegative audience could monitor and adjust their sexual behaviours. Kagan (2018) terms this return to the discourses and anxieties of the early years of the pandemic "a re-crisis" (133). He notes that, in a re-crisis, the boundaries of good and bad sexual behaviour are redrawn in a manner that affirms a neoliberal ideal of health.

de Beistegui (2018, 210–11) defines neoliberalism as an economic system which makes each of us responsible for our own "human capital," thereby stressing the responsibility of the individual over that of the state in the care of people. Under neoliberalism, health becomes both a moral imperative and a "disciplinary rubric" (Dean 2009, 62). As such, maintaining one's seronegative status becomes an exercise in personal responsibility. Race (2001) notes that this neoliberal moralisation of health is partly responsible for the post-crisis "resurgence of blame discourses" (169) concerning the sexual behaviour of gay men.

Alien Sex Club undoubtedly reflected a neoliberal approach to HIV as it focused exclusively on personal risk and behavioural modification. Although the report that inspired the exhibition noted that HIV prevalence in England was at its highest in underprivileged areas of the country (Aghaizu et al. 2013, 24), social inequities, class dynamics and

[8] In 1986, American Journalist William F. Buckley Jr. (1986) wrote in the *New York Times* that "everyone detected with AIDS should be tattooed in the upper forearm, to protect common-needle users, and on the buttocks, to prevent the victimization of other homosexuals." Dan Brouwer (1998) wrote about the HIV/AIDS tattoos in the 1980s and 1990s as a process "of self-stigmatization" where "marking of oneself as "tainted" operated as a "communicative and performative strategy grounded in visibility politics and practised in the context of AIDS activism" (115). The ritualised stigmatisation of the bug chaser in Walter's painting harks back to these early discourses on HIV and visibility, as the tattoos are centred on making seropositivity legible through the body.

governmental responsibilities were largely ignored. This neoliberal perspective on sex, risk and HIV is visualised in the exhibition's recurrent use—and juxtaposition of—the maze and the labyrinth.

Walter (2016, 209) explains that he wanted to establish a contrast between the spatial metaphors of the maze and the labyrinth. He notes,

> A maze is a multi-pronged path that encourages getting lost whilst a labyrinth is a single path that is designed for meditation [...] I returned to the idea that if the cruise maze was an inherently risk-prone space then perhaps the labyrinth was a kind of spatial prophylactic—a sort of architectural version of Pre-Exposure Prophylaxis. This distinction between the maze and labyrinth becomes a leitmotif of the installation.

Walter saw the maze as signifying the risky and irrational activity of purposefully getting lost, a sentiment repeated in his description of cruising as a "dangerous casting off of self" (129). The labyrinth, by comparison, is associated with self-care and rationality: one cannot stray from the path or recklessly abandon oneself within its walls.

In *He is Suffering Because He Has Burned Out the Dopamine Receptors in His Brain* (2013–2014), a disembodied head, pictured with a dense maze for a brain, cries in open-mouthed anguish as tears spurt onto the pages of what could be a diary. Likewise, in *He is Trapped in an Adrenalin Maze* (2013–2014), the maze is presented as a trap locking the cruiser in a biochemical thrall. This marrying of queer promiscuity with addiction is also evident in Todd's (2016) book *Straight Jacket: How to be Gay and Happy.*[9] Like Walter, Todd employs a biological model of addiction in his book, referring to medical studies that show "[...] the brain on cocaine and the brain when sexually aroused are virtually indistinguishable" as proof of the corrupting power of sex. He likens Grindr to a "drug" and a "poison" (216), one that will necessitate some readers to attend "a Sex and Love Addicts meeting" (313). Dean (2015) argues that, in the con-

[9] A former editor of the British gay lifestyle magazine *Attitude*, Todd believed that "the normalization of extreme sex culture" and the continued existence of gay saunas had a causal relationship with "worryingly high levels of sexually transmitted infections, including HIV" (315). Sporting a striking testimonial from Elton John on its essentiality "for every gay person on the planet," the book's blurb claims to offer gay men a way through "depression, drug abuse and sex addiction" so they can "finally get the lives they really want" (2018). As with *Alien Sex Club,* Todd's book is undergirded by neoliberal rationalities as it is chiefly through modifications to the self that gay men can overcome shame, rooted in a history of homophobia.

text of subcultural or extreme sexual practices, addiction often feels like the only valid explanation for "[...] what from a rationalist perspective appears as the inexplicable abdication of self-interest" (235). Therefore, in Walter's art and Todd's writing, sex is a dangerous agentic entity, one that can rob gay men of their sovereignty as rational neoliberal subjects.

In *The History of Sexuality*, Foucault (1978) insists that if we want to "counter the grips of power," then "[i]t is the agency of sex that we must break away from" (157). Sex should be—as Jagose (2012) explains—something we *have* rather "than something that has us" (189). However, neoliberal-inflected moral panics reinvest in the agency of sex, invoking the anxiety-inducing spectre of Rubin's (1984) "erotic DMZ" (282) in the process. Once again, queer sex is pathologised as deviant, harmful and excessive, as something to be monitored and controlled lest it break free and wreak havoc on self and society. Re-crisis discourses on queer sex exert a hauntological force on the past, as well as the present. In constructing the cruiser as a symbol of anachronism and risk, the sexual past emerges in *Alien Sex Club* as an abject temporal space, one that sits in opposition to the progressive 'good gay' behaviour of neoliberal rationality and self-management. Although unintentional, by focusing on personal responsibility and regressive behaviours, *Alien Sex Club* reinforces a harmful narrative about HIV/AIDS: that gay men's promiscuity was somehow responsible for the genesis of the pandemic. It is this warping of the sexual past and the associated narrative of culpability that Castiglia and Reed (2012) attempt to contest and remedy in their book on HIV and cultural memory.

5.3 Who Does Memory Serve?

In *If Memory Serves*, Castiglia and Reed (2012) refer to a shame-laden reading of the sexual past as "unremembering" (10). In unremembering, the sexual cultures of the pre-AIDS years are not erased outright. Instead, they are recollected as abject and anachronistic; as something that defines the limit of progressive, contemporary gay identity. The authors take issue with this turn away from the past and the elision of the positive and life-affirming aspects of these sexual subcultures. Namely, how they cultivated the "systems of cultural communication and care" (23) that were vital for supporting a community in crisis. Like viral hauntology, Freccero's (2006) work on queer spectrality examines how past events can reverberate through time, irrupting in the present as a pressing command or "ethical imperative" (Dinshaw et al. 2007, 184). In Castiglia and Reed's (2012) case, the ghostly voids in an unremembered past issue a call to action: they feel compelled to intervene and offer a way to repair this fissure in cultural memory. Their central thesis is that memory can be redemptive: it can dismantle the narrative of culpability that blamed gay men for the pandemic. Advocating for "strategic remembering" (10), the authors insist that privileging memories that affirm contemporary gay identity offers a way to transform the present and heal a community and past fractured by AIDS.

Many scholars have explored how retrospection and nostalgia can be instrumental in inspiring political action and idealism in the present (Hilderbrand 2006; Muñoz 2009; Shahani 2012). However, Castiglia and Reed's (2012) theorisation of reparative memory is hindered by reductive, gay exceptionalism. In their text, strategic remembering is ethically pure and innately political: "an act of resistance, regardless of its content" (11). Yet, processes of repair are not outside the lines of power they interrogate and contest. Although queer reparative critique is associated with Eve Kosofsky Sedgwick (2003), Carolyn Laubender (2019) traces its theoretical origins in the paediatric-focused literature of psychoanalyst Melanie Klein. Laubender highlights that, for Klein, "reparation names the child's phantasy not necessarily the object's need" (57). While enacting repair might flood the child with a sense of "ethical action," this righteous feeling is unconnected "with the status of the object as the (potentially unwilling) recipient of such assignations of injury and repair" (53). Most critically then, this presumption of ethical action obscures how reparative processes can reaffirm "circuits of violence" (57): attempts at repairing the past can also cause harm and yield their own forms of unremembering.

This critique is true of *If Memory Serves*, as evidenced in the authors' criticism of *The Memorial to Homosexuals Persecuted Under Nazism* (2008), a monument which sits at the outer bounds of the *Tiergarten*, a park in Berlin. Designed by the artistic duo Michael Elmgreen and Ingar Dragset, the structure consists of a single concrete stele canted at an angle, with a small head-height opening on this side. Peering through this gap allows a lone viewer to see an endlessly looping video inside. At the monument's initial unveiling, the black and white footage depicted two men passionately kissing in the *Tiergarten*. Although the structure was intended to memorialise the historical persecution of homosexuals, Haakenson (2010) highlights how the monument's collapsing of the "visible and knowable" with the "secretive and hidden" also raises questions on "the contemporary acceptance of homosexuality" (146). The immediate vandalism of the structure in 2008, and again in 2019 (Greenberger 2019), gives credence to Haakenson's point about queer people's continued fractious relationship with the public realm. Despite the nuanced interweaving of historical and contemporary queer visibility presented by the artwork, Castiglia and Reed (2012) criticised Elmgreen and Dragset's monument for alluding to the practice of cruising. They insisted that idealising "the stealth homosexual, who cruises parks and back alleys undetected, is to valorise an image of the queer as loner or as victim, as in flight from or trapped by a stigmatized identity" (87). Their description of the cruiser painted an image of a shameful anachronism: a shadowy figure limned in the dim light of the closet. In framing the men in the film "as hidden, isolated, and subject to a peeping gaze" (89), the monument seemed to reify "a pulling back from spatial visibility that paralleled calls for the de-generational unremembering of a diseased lifestyle" (90–91). In the authors' eyes, the monument squandered an opportunity to create an unmistakably gay *lieux de mémoire*: a structure that spoke to and represented "an identity constructed in the present in relation to the past" (91).[10] The snatched intimacies and shadowy haunts of the cruiser were disavowed because they clashed discordantly with the idealised image of gay identity the authors wanted to affirm, one grounded in the positive qualities of pride, visibility, and community.

Both Phelan (2010) and Joseph (2002) provide potent critiques of the uncritical valorisation of community, noting that it tends to cultivate an exclusionary identity grounded in capitalist consumption rather than shared political aspirations. Castiglia and Reed's (2012) approach to gay cultural memory is hampered by similar identitarian limitations as it constricts cultural memory around a historically contingent, ideal form of gay identity. Therefore, post-crisis reparative memory projects, even avowedly anti-homonormative ones, can erase, exclude and *unremember* aspects of the past in their efforts to redeem denigrated practices and identities. Leo Bersani (1987) alluded to this in the early years of the pandemic when he described "a frenzied epic of displacement in the discourse on sexuality" (220). In the face of homophobic AIDS rhetoric, gay cruising cultures were often memorialised as utopic "Whitmanesque" (206) democracies of

[10] French historian Pierre Nora described a *lieu de mémoire* as "any significant entity, whether material or nonmaterial in nature" that becomes "a symbolic element of the memorial heritage of any community" (Nora and Kritzman 1996, xvii).

unparalleled "diversity and pluralism" (220). Despite Bersani's warnings against formulating "lost bathhouses as laboratories of ethical liberalism" (222), many post-crisis texts have continued this intellectual investment in the political potency and ethical superiority of queer sex. For example, in the canonical text *Times Square Red, Times Square Blue*, Delany (1999) argues that sex between men in erotic theatres facilitated a vital form of 'interclass contact'. However, Stuelke's (2021) analysis of Delany's accounts of sex with poor and homeless men critiques the author for eroticising, rather than interrogating, the inequities generated by a racial capitalist system. She points out that Delany presents "cross-racial, cross-class sexual contact as the ultimate act and end of solidarity" (62) without ever showing how interclass contact benefits the individual of lower social standing.

In a similar vein to Delany, Dean (2009) theorises street cruising as a virtuous practice, one that cultivates an "ethical philosophy of living" (5) due to its inherent openness to strangers. More recently, Roach (2021) argues that digital cruising on the location-based hook-up app Grindr holds a potent "ethical promise" (48) as its digital affordances *might* train users "to relate in ways that exceed neoliberal aims" (26). These queer texts all seek to affirm the value of cruising cultures by foregrounding their ethicopolitical potential. However, the net effect is that queer impersonal intimacies are idealised as being more radical, political or ethical than 'regular' heteronormative ones.

Jagose (2012) and Amin (2017) write about the tendency in queer scholarship to concentrate on dissident and marginal sexual practices as objects of reparative investment. Amin (2017), in particular, highlights the hauntological dimensions of this redemptive impulse, arguing that the vocal valorisation of queer sexual practices is a direct response to a "damaging legacy of shame and stigma" (6). Moral panics that stigmatise and denigrate queer sexuality and sociality should undoubtedly be divested of their disciplinary power. Yet, as Jagose (2012) explains, reparative theory that valorises the "political potential of subcultural sexual practices" (188) simply inverts Rubin's (1984) hierarchy to establish the value and importance of queer sociosexual practices. This is certainly the case in Moore's (2004) reparative text, *Beyond Shame: Reclaiming the Abandoned History of Radical Gay Sexuality*. Moore's book is an anti-homonormative polemic that attempts to foster pride for a time when gay men were "the creative vanguard of American life"—a time when their sexual exploits were so creative, he sees them as constituting "art" (78). Moore had noble intentions of redeeming the 1970s sexual subcultures once cast as the "abattoirs of the epidemic" (Sullivan 2014, 45). However, in rhapsodising New York cruising clubs as sites of radical social transformation, Moore's nostalgia for the sexual past warps the memory of these spaces into a restrictive masculinist phantasy.

5.4 Nostalgia and *Beyond Shame*

While New York City has a long and rich history of cruising (Chauncey 1995; Turner 2003), the 1970s was a particularly fertile period for the public sex cultures of the city. Men cruised the collapsing piers and empty warehouses of the New York Waterfront (Anderson 2019; Weinberg 2019), casual intimacies sparked in backrooms and bathhouses (Bérubé 2003), and spaces like *The Mineshaft* (Tattelman 2005; Brodsky 1993) catered to a burgeoning sadism and masochism (S&M) scene. However, in the 1980s and 1990s, many of these spaces closed, both due to the AIDS pandemic (Engel and Lyle 2017) and the urban redevelopment of the city (Warner 2000; Ferguson 2018); the latter imposed a heterosexist ideal on the public spaces of the city. The dimming of a once vibrant public sex culture led Douglas Crimp (1989) to remark that, in addition to the loss of life, what many men lost through AIDS was "a culture of sexual possibility" (11). Wayne Hoffman (1996) described this cultural reduction as a "sexual devolution": a feeling among young gay men that the pandemic triggered a "narrowing of sexual freedoms, a clamping down on sexual expression, a withering of sexual worlds" (340). Patrick Moore's book *Beyond Shame* (2004) is, in part, a response to the ostensible de-sexualisation of gay culture in the wake of AIDS.

Originally hailing from Iowa, Moore did not reach the city until a point in the 1980s when much of its legendary sexual cultures seemed to be "in decline and what remained was joyless" (xxii–xxiii). Believing vital portions of the gay past were "being lost or wilfully abandoned" (xxii), Moore's book *Beyond Shame* aimed to reanimate the creative spirit of New York's gay subcultures and push back against their unremembering. As Jose Esteban Muñoz (2009) points out, New York's 'lost' sexual cultures "never completely ceased to be" (33): they persisted—albeit in muted, less tangible forms—through the crisis years and continue to inspire and inform queer culture today. However, this narrative of loss and cultural eradication is a potent one. It exerts a hauntological force that issues a cultural imperative to preserve "its memory, its ghosts, and the ritualized performances of transmitting its vision of utopia across generational divides" (34). This reaction to loss, where there is a movement from "deprivation to vision," is referred to as "melancholic ideality" (Castiglia and Reed 2012, 182). In melancholic ideality, loss is generative: memory fragments and traces of the past are catalysed into hopes and aspirations for the present and future.

This productive approach to loss is rooted in Agambenian melancholia. In *Stanzas* (1993), Agamben introduces the medieval phenomenon of "the Noonday Demon" (3–5), a condition afflicting cloistered monks. Here, the melancholic turns away from the present and "plunges into exaggerated praise of distant and absent monasteries," evoking all the "places where he could be healthy and happy" among "pleasant communities of brothers" (4). Castiglia and Reed (2012) point out that Agambenian melancholy revolves around a phantasmatic ideal rather than a lost object since "the beloved, being ideal, has never been possessed and therefore cannot be lost" (181). Therefore, unlike Freudian melancholia, where "the grieving subject" staves off a loss by internalising "residues of the lost object" (Min 2003, 232), Agambenian melancholia allows "loss and idealism" (Castiglia and Reed 2012, 179) to operate in tandem. Castiglia and Reed (2012) suggest that this yearning for a (wholly imagined) better time and place aligns with a queer "phantasmatic ideal of sexual subculture" (182). However, they stress that such phantasmatic investments are not nostalgic attempts to restore cruising cultures to their former glory. Instead, cultural investment in a lost sexual past is a "seedbed of inventive idealization" (193) that inspires people "to envision and protect new ideals" (183).

Moore's melancholic attachment to 1970s gay sexual culture is undeniable: he drapes it "in the funereal garb of loss" (Castiglia and Reed 2012, 182), stating that "as a gay man who missed those years [he refuses] to abandon their memory" (Moore 2004, xxv). His book is intended as a clarion call for a new generation, an insistence that they continue the "great social experiment initiated by gay men using their bodies and sexual creativity," something he believes was "the true sexual revolution" (4). While this corporeal celebration might appear like melancholic ideality—cruising memories inspiring political idealism in the present—Moore (2004) falls into the trap of reactively idealising certain gay sexual subcultures as uniquely radical and transformative. In *Beyond Shame*, defunct New York sex clubs are not sites of sexual sociality or queer culture; through Moore's lionisation, they become harbingers of a "social change" that match "the more radical elements of that era's anti-war, civil rights, and feminist movements" (xxiv). AIDS truncated their "astonishing experiment," which, Moore attests, "might have transformed America by creating entirely new models of sexual interaction" (4).

However, as Patricia Stuelke (2021) notes, reparative attempts to celebrate the queer past often position "the world-making project of surviving within homophobic capitalist heteroculture" as being equal "with changing the world, even as it does not bring an end to capitalism and empire" (149). Therefore, in casting sex clubs as incubators for groundbreaking change, Moore forges an idealised and false connection between gay sex and political power. While sex clubs were valuable strategic spatial productions, they did not—and still do not—have world-changing agency. They may feel emancipatory and revelatory, but they are not revolutionary.

Moore's phantasy of radical political eros is centred on an ideal image of hypermasculine gay sex clubs. One that creates a "living-up-to-them dynamic" (Dean 2009, 23) for a time when gay men had the "courageous willingness to risk absolutely everything" (Moore 2004, xxv) for their desires.[11] To him, sex in these spaces was not sociable, playful or pleasurable: it was a deadly serious ritual undertaken by "grim-faced men who knew in their hearts that they were embarking on a journey from which they might never return" (Moore 2004, 23). Whereas in *Alien Sex Club*, sexual risk was cast as an abdication of personal responsibility, here Moore inverts this association. Self-abnegation is lauded as exemplary, thereby transmuting the leather-clad men of *The Mineshaft* into—potentially unwilling—martyrs to sexual radicalism. Instead of uncoupling them from moralising narratives of self-harm and personal destruction, Moore merely romanticises and mythologises 'risky' sexual practices.

In his writing on white gay masculinity, Halberstam (2005) notes that shame operates as "a gendered form of sexual abjection: it belongs to the feminine, and when men find themselves 'flooded' with shame, chances are they are being feminized in some way and against their will" (226). Gay shame, in this case, is grounded in the ignominy of being emasculated and denied one's expected patriarchal dividend. The gendered dynamics of shame are evident in Moore's argumentative line as he equates the

[11] In *Manhood and Politics*, Wendy Brown (1988) states that the "historical symbiosis of courage and manliness" is based on a "willingness to risk death for an abstract aim" (206). Therefore, "courage," for a man, is indelibly linked to "overcoming bodily fears and overcoming concerns for life" (206).

feminisation of queer culture to its desexualisation. He baulks at the popularity of drag, stating that in "fifty years' time we will look back at drag and camp as the minstrel shows of gay culture—amusing but ultimately sinister and degrading, an easy way for straight culture to avoid the realities of our sexuality" (Moore 2004, 120). Moore's attempt to repair gay culture's position as "a community of shame" (xxi) is arguably centred on salvaging a particular form of cis gay masculinity so cultural memory can be repaired into an "uncastrated, muscular, whole" (Halberstam 2005, 228) in the process. Therefore, *Beyond Shame* is grounded in an unproductive form of nostalgia, one that reactively idealises a narrow, masculinist phantasy of the sexual past.

In *The Future of Nostalgia*, Svetlana Boym (2008) makes a distinction between restorative and reflective nostalgia. Whereas reflective nostalgia thrives in loss and "longing," restorative nostalgia "attempts a transhistorical reconstruction of the lost home" through arguments for "truth and tradition" (xviii). The central issue with restorative nostalgia is that the past is no longer "a duration but a perfect snapshot" (49). This is redolent of Walter Benjamin's (1989) description of historicism as the work of historians who wish "to relive an era," an approach that ultimately results in *acedia* as they fruitlessly grasp onto a brief "historical image" (257). Moore's communion with the sexual past can be understood as a nostalgic act of restorative historicism as he crafts a—wholly unreal—phantasy image of a radical sexual utopia.

Much like Castiglia and Reed's (2012) approach to cultural memory is built on the reification of an ideal form of gay political identity, *Beyond Shame*'s restorative nostalgia ossifies the sexual past into a golden ideal that smooths out the elements that do not fit its romanticising narrative of masculine gay communion. Where John Walter's *Alien Sex Club* forged a totemic image of the sexual past as a lapsarian site of risky behaviour, Moore's book merely inverts, rather than interrogates, this association. Gay men become noble risk-takers in the pursuit of an undefined radical goal. In both cases, memories of the past are constricted into flat, simplistic narratives in the service of neoliberal or masculinist rhetoric. However, by examining the collaborative artist book project *Petite Mort*, this chapter proposes a deidealising approach to the sexual past, one that reflects on memories of public sex without idealising the practice of cruising.

5.5 Deidealisation and *Petite Mort*

Petite Mort: Recollections of a Queer Public (2011) is a collaborative artist book project co-curated by Ingrid Chu and Savannah Gorton, commissioned for the curatorial initiative Forever & Today. Devised as "an atlas of queer affection" (7) by invited artist Carlos Motta in collaboration with scholar Joshua Lubin-Levy, *Petite Mort* brings together an intergenerational group of over 60 contributors who submitted drawings from memory of their public sex experiences in New York City.

In flicking through its pages, one is struck by the distinct lack of figuration in the works; the memories seem to cohere around city spaces rather than sexual acts or people. There are drawings of empty rooftops and city streets, vacant shipping terminals and subway stops, dimly lit toilets and darkrooms. However, the emptiness and simplicity of these images do not trigger a nostalgic or mournful feeling of loss. The viewer knows these pictures are memory traces of sex in public, and the ghostly unseen presence/absence of those sexual encounters imbue the sprawling rooftops and city streets with yearning and anticipatory energy.

An example is Antoine Vigne 2011 in Motta and Lubin-Levy (2011) memory (Fig. 5.1)—sketched with the help of artist Daniel-Greenfield Campoverde—of being cruised by a man as he walked to work. The vantage point of the picture offers an expansive view of the street as the text descends from the horizon, a space which is metaphorically bound, within queer theory, to potentiality and ideality (Muñoz 2009). Images like Vigne's—where nondescript urban spaces are suffused with individuals' memories of queer public intimacy—offer a perspective on *lieux de mémoire*, which is individual and collective rather than communal or cultural.

Through a reading of Kathryn Bond Stockton's (2009) work on queer childhoods, Castiglia and Reed (2012) insist that memory can "enlarge the present" (12–13), enriching it with the feelings and pleasures of the past. This is precisely what we see in Vigne's drawing: it is a moment where the fabric of the heteronormative world rips to reveal a queer one glittering just beneath its surface. For Vigne, this clandestine encounter reshapes his relation to this quotidian space: it now carries spectral traces of this erotic experience.

Artist George Towne 2011 in Motta and Lubin-Levy (2011) watercolour painting of a gay adult video store in the East Village also affirms this connection between queerness and public space. After moving to the city

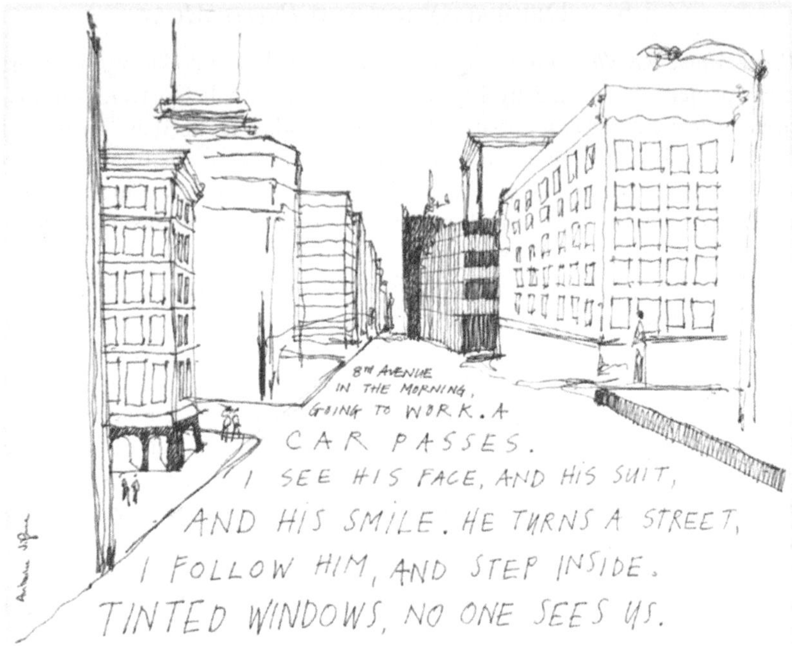
8TH AVENUE
IN THE MORNING,
GOING TO WORK. A
CAR PASSES.
I SEE HIS FACE, AND HIS SUIT,
AND HIS SMILE. HE TURNS A STREET,
I FOLLOW HIM, AND STEP INSIDE.
TINTED WINDOWS, NO ONE SEES US.

Fig. 5.1 Antoine Vigne and Daniel-Greenfield Campoverde, *8th Avenue* (2011)

in 1986, Towne regularly passed this store and would later establish a long-term friendship with a man he met there following "a night of bar-hopping" (76). Towne explains that this shop was one of the few visibly gay spaces in the city: it "made me feel good, as it validated my existence" (76). In both cases, *Petite Mort* demonstrates how memories of public sex can innervate everyday space with meanings and feelings that sustain queer subjects as they move through a heterosexist world.

Although many of the images in *Petite Mort*—such as Vigne's above—are undated, the ones that are establish a timeline running from the 1970s to 2010. When viewed in concert, these memories do not establish a golden age of cruising or a clear demarcation before and after AIDS. Instead, they form a gestalt mnemonic entity, an intergenerational *archive of feelings* (Cvetkovich 2003), that registers subjective accounts and fragmentary memories of public sex in the city. An example is Seth Joseph Weine's contribution, entitled *Hole in my Heart* (Fig. 5.2), where he meditates on his experiences in the city's gay saunas over the previous 35 years.

The image consists of text arranged in a heart shape, containing within an aerial view of a spare bathhouse cubicle with an open door and a narrow bed. In the text, Weine recalls an impactful encounter with a handsome man in the intense heat of a sauna. The memory of their sweat-slicked bodies remains "one of the high points in [his] eros seeking life" (2011, 131). However, towards the end of his drawing, he admits that in his last few years of attending these spaces, he started to feel ill at ease and ultimately left "feeling emptied rather than fulfilled" (131). Whereas Vigne's drawing carries glimmers of queer utopianism, Weine's memories are marked by a feeling of ambivalence. He may have had exciting experiences in cruising spaces, but he also remembers a gnawing feeling of emptiness.

Another contributor, Michael, submitted a detailed sketch of the interior of an empty New York cab interior with a string of rowhouse stoops just legible through the driver's window. In the short text accompanying his drawing, Michael recounts that a few years previous, he had sex with a taxi driver because he "was pretty down about a guy and life and being twenty-four" but admitted the encounter "didn't really help" (114). Jagose (2012) argues that when the impersonal intimacies that arise from subaltern sexual practices are exceptionalised as radical and liberatory, they become "folded back into personalizing models of selfhood" (188). That is, if heteronormativity assures fulfilment through the cultivation of deep personal connections, and anti-normative sexual discourses merely invert this association, then impersonal intimacy becomes a route to a good queer life. Despite their age difference, there is a sense of continuity between Michael and Weine's experiences in that queer dissident sex does not fulfil or affirm either party. Neither man offers an idealised account of cruising; instead, their memories stress the plurality of subjective experience.

Cruising spaces have always been polysemic zones of queer contact. People explore sexual identities and subjectivities in these spaces, while others might want to suspend or forget them. These can be spaces of pleasure and queer communion, but they can also be laced with feelings of fear, confusion and shame. The chapter illustrates that ignoring the contradictory complexity of cruising cultures yields simplified narratives of shameful pre-liberatory invisibility, infection risk and bold sexual radicalism. However, unlike *Beyond Shame*, *Alien Sex Club* or *If Memory Serves*, *Petite Mort* does not offer a "totalizing narrative" (Motta and Lubin-Levy

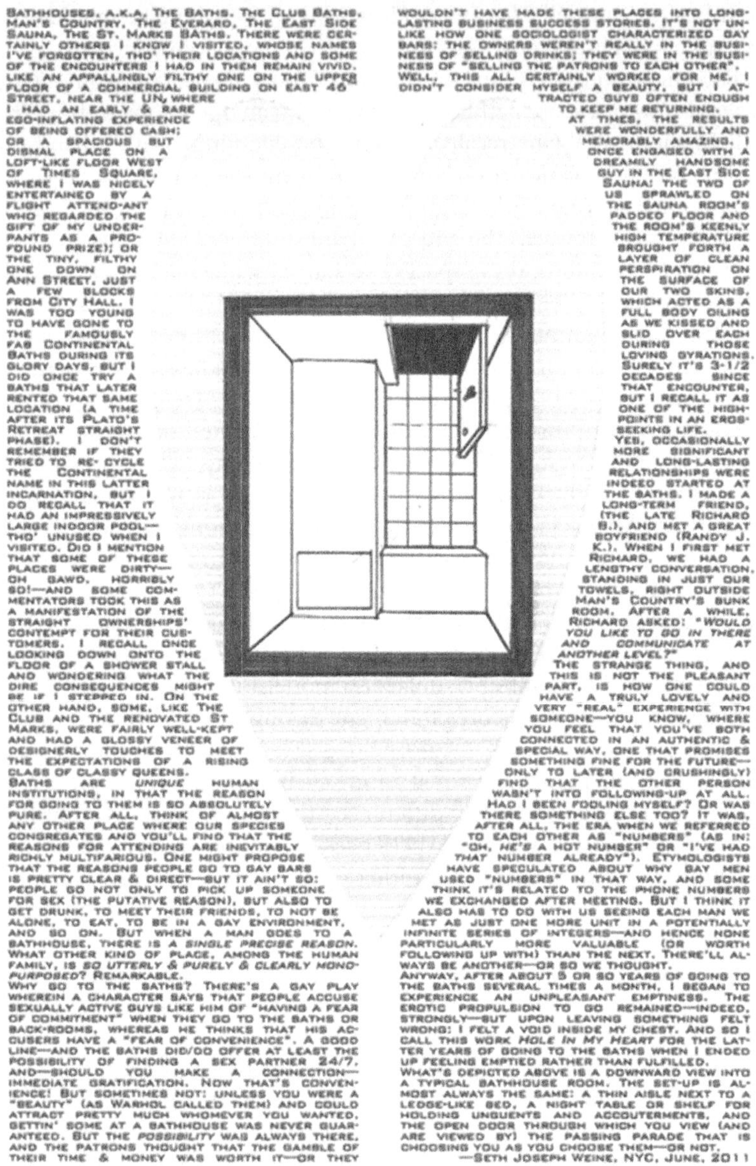

Fig. 5.2 Seth Joseph Weine, *Hole in My Heart* (2011)

2011, 12) of public sex. As seen in the drawings which are discussed above, the collaborative artist book holds space for ambivalent feelings and perspectives that do not cohere around an ideal image of liberatory queer sex.

Cruising, in *Petite Mort*, is not a radical appropriation of public space, a form of political visibility or a generative route to community. Instead, it emerges as a practice that is, at once, furtive and brazen, solitary and collective, a way to find and escape oneself. The plurality and diversity of its memories establishes a sense of individualised collectivity that is redolent of French philosopher Jean-Luc Nancy's (2000) concept of "being singular plural." Rather than binding public sex to a shared identity, a cultural inheritance or an established community, *Petite Mort* underscores how a desire for connection and a longing to be seen resounds through all human experience.

Following the contributors' memory drawings, *Petite Mort* contains a series of short written pieces from 12 queer academics and writers—including John Paul Ricco, Kate Bornstein and Jose Esteban Muñoz—who were asked to give a short response to the question 'Does Public Sex Matter?' Although Muñoz in *Cruising Utopia* (2009) argued that public sex cultures held the blueprints "for actual, living sexual citizenship" (35), his response to the question demonstrates a deidealising shift. He admitted that his previous writing on public sex had been "too celebratory, too ecstatic" (2011, 155). Now, he is unsure of the worth of casting "the bright of publicity" on public sex, given it often emphasises an idealised image of a "liberated gay man" (155) who boldly challenges hetero/homonormativity with each sexual act. Instead, Muñoz insists that:

> The time has come to understand public sex as an unshareable thing that queers manage to share. But the sharing needs to resist the impulse towards ecstatic celebration, romantic remembrance, and spectacle. Maybe it's enough to know public sex simply matters and to practice resisting the impulse to pull it apart and put it on display. Let us be content to share the fact of the unsharable (155).

As already discussed, the neoliberal-inflected panic discourses apparent in *Alien Sex Club* undoubtedly pull cruising apart and turn it into an abject spectacle. However, in the extract above, Muñoz suspects that queer investments in the radicalism of cruising expose it in the same way.

This is something that this chapter has explored: in the post-crisis era, the hauntological imperative to protect subcultural sexual practices sees them swaddled in the language of revolutionary power and ethical possibility. Yet, theorising queer sex as speaking "in the tongue of liberation" (Jagose 2012, 2) requires it to be rigorously dissected for proof of its radicalism. If Foucault's (1978) work demonstrated that connecting sex to an inner truth allowed it to become enmeshed with biopower, then siting a kernel of ethicopolitcal potentiality within non-normative sexual behaviours risks reinstating the same epistemological imperative around sex. That is, anti-homonormative texts that argue queer sex is "legitimately associated with the honour of a political cause" (6) reaffirm and remain trapped in the discursive machinations of sexuality. Therefore, the idealisation of queer sex not only affirms the Rubinesque value system, it also bolsters a "will to knowledge" (12) with respect to sexuality.

The belief that queer sex—once regarded as deviant and dangerous—is a generative tool for social and political change transmutes historical shame and ignominy into something affirming and inspiring in the present. Yet, idealising queer sex in this manner places it on a tottering pedestal: there is no way for it to "fulfil the outsized hopes we invest in [it]" (Amin 2017, 108). If we want to embrace and understand "the variegated textures of queer," then we need "to deidealize the queer imaginaries we treasure the most" (175). Deidealisation "means learning to live with rather than redeem or critique the imperfect and messy relations" (79) borne from a turbulent past. It means not continuing the "frenzied epic of displacement in the discourse on sexuality" (Bersani 1987, 220) by loading queer sex with further agency and meaning.

In creating a multi-perspective, intergenerational memory project, *Petite Mort* is a perfect example of deidealisation in practice. It does not attempt to create a cohesive idea of cruising in the city, one that affirms a positive image of queer radicalism. Instead, it embraces the inherent spectrality of the past, accepting rather than disavowing its complexities, contradictions and "queer impurities" (Amin 2017, 175). Unlike the other artefacts examined, it learns "to live *with* ghosts" (Derrida 1994, xvii–xviii, emphasis in original) rather than banishing them away or *puppetting* them in the service of homonormative, neoliberal or anti-normative discourses.

Gay politics has adopted several defensive strategies in a bid to affirm and authenticate gay existence. The biological essentialism of 'Born This Way' insists that gay people should not face oppression because they do not have the agency to choose their desires. The myth of the "eternal homosexual" (D'Emilio 2007)—the political argument that gay people deserve equality and freedom from persecution due to their presence "throughout history, in all societies and all periods" (250–51)—mounts a similar defence, albeit grounded in historical, rather than biological, essentialism. Writing on these political strategies, Shah (1998) argues that we should not need to hunt for historical origins "to sanction our existence"; what matters is that queer people exist right now; "on that alone we demand acknowledgement and acceptance" (148–49). The same is true of a subcultural practice like cruising: it does not need to generate novel social structures, ethics or radical politics for it to be culturally important or of personal value.

Queer sexual subcultures have been interrogated and undermined through state-mandated homophobia, medical taxonomies, theories of deviance, and neoliberal-informed arguments on sexual excess. Understandably, the hauntological impact of the AIDS crisis and a history of homophobic oppression generate an imperative to preserve and defend these vilified practices. Yet, queer people have spent far too long confessing and defending their desires. There is power in refusing to qualify them within a hierarchy of good and bad behaviours, in refusing to provide evidence of their generative value.

Muñoz (2011) states that maybe it is "enough to know public sex simply matters" (155). To develop his point, cruising matters because it *feels* like it matters. In the face of viral hauntology, there is a self-determining power in concentrating on the intensity and complexity of the feelings cruising inspires, rather than burdening it with the responsibility of realising queer utopia and revolutionary change. Part of this discursive investment in cruising has been to offset its ephemerality, to give it the same importance and futurity afforded to heteronormative intimacies. Yet, cruising's value lies in revelation, not revolution. That brief encounter on the street—the knowing backward glance, its pressure lingering in memory—can feel like a fracturing moment, one where the fabric of the heteronormative world rips to reveal a queer one glimmering just beneath its surface. These snatched intimacies might flash in and out of being, but the complex feelings they inspire—desire, excitement, trepidation, shame—have spun myriad inchoate life-worlds into being. As a way of seeing and being seen, cruising ruptures the present, tilting our gaze onto queer vistas undulating with feeling, meaning and desire.

References

Agamben, Giorgio. 1993. *Stanzas: Word and Phantasm in Western Culture.* Minneapolis: University of Minnesota Press.

Aghaizu, A., A.E. Brown, A. Nardone, O. Gill, and V. Delpech. 2013. *HIV in the United Kingdom 2013 Report: Data to End 2012.* London: Public Health England.

Amin, Kadji. 2017. *Disturbing Attachments: Genet, Modern Pederasty, and Queer History.* Durham: Duke University Press.

Anderson, Fiona. 2019. *Cruising the Dead River: David Wojnarowicz and New York's Ruined Waterfront.* Chicago: University of Chicago Press.

Benjamin, Walter. 1989. Theses on the Philosophy of History. In *Critical Theory and Society A Reader*, 255–263. New York: Routledge.

Bersani, Leo. 1987. Is the Rectum a Grave? *October* 43: 197–222. https://doi.org/10.2307/3397574.

Bérubé, Allan. 2003. The History of Gay Bathhouses. *Journal of Homosexuality* 44 (3–4): 33–53.

Boym, Svetlana. 2008. *The Future of Nostalgia.* Hachette UK.

Brodsky, Joel I. 1993. The Mineshaft: A Retrospective Ethnography. *Journal of Homosexuality* 24 (3–4): 233–252. https://doi.org/10.1300/J082v24n03_16.

Brouwer, Dan. 1998. The Precarious Visibility Politics of Self-Stigmatization: The Case of HIV/AIDS Tattoos. *Text and Performance Quarterly* 18 (2): 114–136. https://doi.org/10.1080/10462939809366216.

Brown, Wendy. 1988. *Manhood and Politics: A Feminist Reading in Political Theory.* Totowa: Rowman & Littlefield.

———. 2001. *Politics Out of History.* Princeton: Princeton University Press.

Buckley Jr., William F. 1986. Crucial Steps in Combating the AIDS Epidemic: Identify All the Carriers. *New York Times* 18: A27.

Castiglia, Christopher, and Christopher Reed. 2012. *If Memory Serves: Gay Men, AIDS, and the Promise of the Queer Past.* Minneapolis: University of Minnesota Press.

Chauncey, George. 1995. *Gay New York: The Making of the Gay Male World, 1890-1940.* London: Flamingo.

Creed, Barbara. 1993. *The Monstrous-Feminine: Film, Feminism, Psychoanalysis.* New York: Routledge.

Crimp, Douglas. 1989. Mourning and Militancy. *October* 51: 3–18. https://doi.org/10.2307/778889.

———. 2002. *Melancholia and Moralism: Essays on AIDS and Queer Politics.* Cambridge: MIT Press.

Cvetkovich, Ann. 2003. *An Archive of Feelings: Trauma, Sexuality, and Lesbian Public Cultures.* Durham: Duke University Press.

Daskalakis, Demetre, Richard Silvera, Kyle Bernstein, Dylan Stein, Robert Hagerty, Richard Hutt, Alith Maillard, William Borkowsky, Judith Aberg, and Fred Valentine. 2009. Implementation of HIV Testing at 2 New York City Bathhouses: From Pilot to Clinical Service. *Clinical Infectious Diseases* 48 (11): 1609–1616.

Dean, Tim. 2009. *Unlimited Intimacy: Reflections on the Subculture of Barebacking*. Chicago: University of Chicago Press.

———. 2015. Mediated Intimacies: Raw Sex, Truvada, and the Biopolitics of Chemoprophylaxis. *Sexualities* 18 (1–2): 224–246.

de Beistegui, Miguel. 2018. *The Government of Desire: A Genealogy of the Liberal Subject*. Chicago: University of Chicago Press.

Delany, Samuel R. 1999. *Times Square Red, Times Square Blue. Sexual Cultures*. New York: New York University Press.

D'Emilio, John. 2007. Capitalism and Gay Identity. In *Culture, Society and Sexuality*, 1st ed. New York: Routledge.

Derrida, Jacques. 1994. *Specters of Marx: The State of the Debt, the Work of Mourning, and the New International*. New York: Psychology Press.

Dinshaw, Carolyn, Lee Edelman, Roderick A. Ferguson, Carla Freccero, Elizabeth Freeman, Judith Halberstam, Annamarie Jagose, Christopher S. Nealon, and Tan Hoang Nguyen. 2007. Theorizing Queer Temporalities: A Roundtable Discussion. *GLQ: A Journal of Lesbian and Gay Studies* 13 (2): 177–195.

Engel, Stephen M., and Timothy S. Lyle. 2017. Fucking with Dignity: Public Sex, Queer Intimate Kinship, and How the AIDS Epidemic Bathhouse Closures Constituted a Dignity Taking. *Chicago-Kent Law Review* 92: 961.

Ferguson, Roderick A. 2018. *One-Dimensional Queer*. Medford: Wiley.

Foucault, Michel. 1978. *The History of Sexuality: An Introduction*. New York: Pantheon Books.

Frank, Katherine. 2019. Rethinking Risk, Culture, and Intervention in Collective Sex Environments. *Archives of Sexual Behavior* 48 (1): 3–30.

Freccero, Carla. 2006. *Queer/Early/Modern*. Durham: Duke University Press.

Gama, Ana, Ana Abecasis, Marta Pingarilho, Luís Mendão, Maria O. Martins, Henrique Barros, and Sónia Dias. 2017. Cruising Venues as a Context for HIV Risky Behavior Among Men Who Have Sex with Men. *Archives of Sexual Behavior* 46 (4): 1061–1068.

Gonzalez, Octavio R. 2019. Pre-Exposure Prophylaxis (PrEP), "the Truvada Whore," and the New Gay Sexual Revolution. *Raw: PrEP, Paedagogy, and the Politics of Barebacking* 47–70.

Greenberger, Alex. 2019. Report: Elmgreen & Dragset's Berlin Monument to Gay Victims of Nazi Persecution Vandalized. *ARTnews.Com* (blog), January 30, 2019. https://www.artnews.com/art-news/news/report-elmgreen-dragsets-berlin-monument-gay-victims-nazi-persecution-vandalized-11808/.

Haakenson, Thomas O. 2010. (In)Visible Trauma: Michael Elmgreen and Ingar Dragset's Memorial to the Homosexuals Persecuted Under the National Socialist Regime. In *Memorialization in Germany Since 1945*, ed. Bill Niven and Chloe Paver, 146–156. London: Palgrave Macmillan UK. https://doi.org/10.1057/9780230248502_14.
Halberstam, Jack. 2005. Shame and White Gay Masculinity. *Social Text* 23 (3–4 (84–85)): 219–233.
Hall, James. 2018. *Dictionary of Subjects and Symbols in Art*. New York: Routledge.
Hilderbrand, Lucas. 2006. Retroactivism. *GLQ: A Journal of Lesbian and Gay Studies* 12 (2): 303–317.
Hoffman, Wayne. 1996. Skipping the Life Fantastic: Coming of Age in the Sexual Devolution. In *Policing Public Sex: Queer Politics and the Future of AIDS Activism*, 337–354. Boston: South End Press.
Jagose, Annamarie. 2012. *Orgasmology*. Durham: Duke University Press.
Joseph, Miranda. 2002. *Against the Romance of Community*. Minneapolis: University of Minnesota Press.
Kagan, Dion. 2018. *Positive Images: Gay Men and HIV/AIDS in the Culture of 'Post Crisis'*. London: Bloomsbury Academic.
Kristeva, Julia. 1982. *Powers of Horror*. Vol. 98. University Presses of California, Columbia and Princeton. http://digitalmedia.arts.ufl.edu/~jack/home/images/archive/6/60/20160825003818%21Kristevapowersofhorrorabjection.pdf.
Laubender, Carolyn. 2019. Beyond Repair: Interpretation, Reparation, and Melanie Klein's Clinical Play-Technique. *Studies in Gender and Sexuality* 20 (1): 51–67. https://doi.org/10.1080/15240657.2019.1559519.
Min, Susette. 2003. Remains to Be Seen: Reading the Works of Dean Sameshima and Khanh Vo. In *Loss: The Politics of Mourning*, ed. David L. Eng and David Kazanjian, 229–250. Berkeley: University of California Press.
Møller, Kristian, and Chase Ledin. 2020. Viral Hauntology: Specters of AIDS in Infrastructures of Gay Sexual Sociability. In *Affects, Interfaces, Events*, ed. B.M. Stavning Thomsen, J. Kofoed, and J. Fritsch. Vancouver: Imbricate!
Moore, Patrick. 2004. *Beyond Shame: Reclaiming the Abandoned History of Radical Gay Sexuality*. Boston: Beacon Press.
Motta, Carlos, and Joshua Lubin-Levy. 2011. *Petite Mort: Recollections of a Queer Public*. New York: Forever & Today. https://carlosmotta.com/project/petite-mort-recollections-of-a-queer-public-2011/.
Muñoz, José Esteban. 2009. *Cruising Utopia: The Then and There of Queer Futurity*. New York: NYU Press.
———. 2011. Sharing Public Sex. In *Petite Mort: Recollections of a Queer Public*, ed. Carlos Motta and Joshua Lubin-Levy. New York: Forever & Today.
Nancy, Jean-Luc. 2000. *Being Singular Plural*. Stanford: Stanford University Press.

Nora, Pierre, and Lawrence D. Kritzman. 1996. *Realms of Memory: Conflicts and Divisions*. New York: Columbia University Press.

Phelan, Shane. 2010. *Sexual Strangers: Gays, Lesbians, and Dilemmas of Citizenship*. Philadelphia: Temple University Press.

Race, Kane. 2001. The Undetectable Crisis: Changing Technologies of Risk. *Sexualities* 4 (2): 167–189. https://doi.org/10.1177/136346001004002004.

Roach, Tom. 2021. *Screen Love: Queer Intimacies in the Grindr Era*. New York: SUNY Press.

Rodger, Alison J., Valentina Cambiano, Tina Bruun, Pietro Vernazza, Simon Collins, Jan van Lunzen, Giulio Maria Corbelli, et al. 2016. Sexual Activity Without Condoms and Risk of HIV Transmission in Serodifferent Couples When the HIV-Positive Partner Is Using Suppressive Antiretroviral Therapy. *JAMA* 316 (2): 171–181. https://doi.org/10.1001/jama.2016.5148.

Rodger, A., V. Cambiano, T. Bruun, P. Vernazza, S. Collins, G.M. Corbelli, O. Degen, et al. 2018. Risk of HIV Transmission through Condomless Sex in MSM Couples with Suppressive ART: The PARTNER2 Study Extended Results in Gay Men. *Journal of the International AIDS Society* 21 (suppl 6): 163–163. https://doi.org/10.1002/jia2.25148.

Rubin, Gayle. 1984. Thinking Sex: Notes for a Radical Theory of the Politics of Sexuality. In *Pleasure and Danger: Exploring Female Sexuality*, ed. Carole S. Vance. New York: Routledge & K. Paul.

Sedgwick, Eve Kosofsky. 2003. *4. Paranoid Reading and Reparative Reading, or, You're So Paranoid, You Probably Think This Essay Is About You*, 123–152. Durham: Duke University Press. https://doi.org/10.1515/9780822384786-007.

Shah, Nayan. 1998. Sexuality, Identity, and the Uses of History. *Q & A: Queer in Asian America* 141–156.

Shahani, Nishant. 2012. *Queer Retrosexualities: The Politics of Reparative Return*. Idaho Falls: Lexington Books.

Stockton, Kathryn Bond. 2009. *The Queer Child, or Growing Sideways in the Twentieth Century*. Durham: Duke University Press.

Stuelke, Patricia. 2021. *The Ruse of Repair: US Neoliberal Empire and the Turn from Critique*. Durham: Duke University Press.

Sullivan, Andrew. 2014. *Love Undetectable: Notes on Friendship, Sex, and Survival*. New York: Knopf Doubleday.

Tattelman, Ira. 2005. Staging Sex and Masculinity at the Mineshaft. *Men and Masculinities* 7 (3): 300–309. https://doi.org/10.1177/1097184X04272120.

Todd, Matthew. 2016. *Straight Jacket*. London: Bantam.

———. 2018. *Straight Jacket: Overcoming Society's Legacy of Gay Shame*. Transworld.

Turner, Mark W. 2003. *Backward Glances: Cruising the Queer Streets of New York and London*. London: Reaktion Books.

Walter, John. 2016. *Alien Sex Club: Educating Audiences About Continuing Rates of HIV Transmission Using Art and Design*. PhD Thesis, University of Westminster.

Warner, Michael. 2000. *The Trouble with Normal: Sex, Politics, and the Ethics of Queer Life*. Cambridge: Harvard University Press.

Watney, Simon. 1987. *Policing Desire: Pornography, AIDS, and the Media*. Madison: University of Minnesota Press.

Weinberg, Jonathan. 2019. *Pier Groups: Art and Sex Along the New York Waterfront*. University Park: Pennsylvania State University Press.

CHAPTER 6

Embodied Topologies: Space and the Place of Memory Among Women Living with HIV in South Africa

Elizabeth Mills

6.1 Remembering the Past and Securing the Future

In 2023, South Africa had the dual distinction of having the world's largest HIV treatment programme and also the highest number of people living with HIV (7.8 million) (Johnson and Dorrington 2023). Stretching back in time to 2010, the successful HIV treatment programme would have been hard to envision as the country emerged from a decade of high-level government denialism of HIV science and a stringent refusal to scale up essential HIV treatment (Simelela et al. 2015, Pillay-van Wyk et al. 2019). Drawing on long-term multi-sited ethnographic research, this chapter centres on the lives of a group of women who had worked as activists to compel the South African government to introduce HIV treatment

E. Mills (✉)
University of Sussex, Brighton, UK
e-mail: E.Mills@sussex.ac.uk

A. Castillo Villanueva, A. Bollas (eds.), *HIV/AIDS in Memory, Culture and Society*, Palgrave Studies in Science and Popular Culture, https://doi.org/10.1007/978-3-031-59699-5_6

in the public health system. Working across three main sections—starting life, life transitions and sustaining life—the chapter recounts women's memories of a time when HIV treatment was unavailable for the majority of South Africans, and it situates these memories in the present through their current experiences of illness, health and hope.

Looking back in time, HIV-positive South Africans were confronted with a new struggle as the country emerged from decades of apartheid and colonialism: the struggle to access HIV treatment (Hodes 2018). Over this time, in the late 1990s and early 2000s, activists and activist organisations like Treatment Action Campaign (TAC) and Medicines Sans Frontiers (MSF) called for epistemological solidarity on the scientific value of HIV medicines as part of a strategy to challenge the AIDS denialism of the government's leaders (including President Thabo Mbeki). The timing of my fieldwork with a group of HIV-positive activists (from 2010 onwards) is significant because it took place on the outer edge of this struggle. While significant, the nature of this research is not new: anthropologists like Fiona Larkin (Larkan et al. 2015, Larkan 2004) and João Biehl have similarly sought to understand how people's memories of HIV (in Brazil and South Africa, respectively) shape their experiences of the present and their perceptions of the future. In my research, I found that by listening to women's accounts of their activism, I was confronted with what Biehl describes as 'the unexpected' (Biehl and Locke 2017; Biehl 2007, 2013). He uses this term to evoke the value of ethnographic research that can move between the past (by understanding memories of illness and the struggle for HIV treatment) and the future (by recognising the power of imagination to open up the horizon of possibility through access to life-extending HIV treatment). In calling for an 'anthropology of becoming', he encourages researchers to engage with 'the unexpected' not simply as an abstract academic principle but as an ethical task: he argues that by thinking beyond the limits of what is perceived to be possible, we call into focus the biomedical horizon of HIV-positive people's future.

In my fieldwork, I encountered 'the unexpected' in two ways. First, I found that the government, under former President Zuma, and activist organisations like TAC had entered a predominantly collaborative rather than combative relationship. This enabled activists, and indeed the government, to shift to a broader recognition of the value of addressing socioeconomic inequalities that undermined the success of the country's ARV programme. As a result, the research upon which this chapter is based explores women's memories and embodied experiences of inequality linked to race, class and gender. In exploring how race, class and gender intersect to create multi-dimensional inequality and undermine health outcomes in South Africa, even in the face of the world's largest ARV rollout, this ethnography tessellates with studies conducted across Sub-Saharan Africa (Wilson and Mapesi 2020; Cancelliere 2020), including in Tanzania (Marsland 2012; Mattes 2019; Nance et al. 2017), Kenya (Prince 2012; Musyoki et al. 2021; Copeland 2018) and Mozambique (Kalofonos 2008; Chapman 2021), that challenge the notion of HIV medical technologies as solely responsible for enabling life (Rose 2006; Young et al. 2019).

While grounded in an understanding of health as it relates to intersectional inequality, this chapter moves out to explore the second unexpected dimension of my ethnographic research. In spending time with women who had fought for HIV treatment in South Africa, I came to understand that memory and place was, for some, far more important for revealing the complexity of their full selves than an excoriation of intersecting 'identities' like HIV, gender, class or race. While women's struggle for a non-projected future continued to be visible in everyday acts like finding food for their child's lunch box or taking their ARVs each evening, it was their memories of earlier lives lived in different places that featured most strongly in their sense-making of their present.

In the sections that follow, I trace the relationship between memory, space and embodiment across these two facets of 'the unexpected' and I suggest that women's memories of what made them who they are shifted depending on where they were located when they shared these recollections with me. Further, I learnt that these memories of different times and shifting spaces were not only held in women's narrative accounts but also in their bodies. I argue that memories and place matter, not only for how they relate to one another but because of how they relate to one another *within* the body. By engaging with political science, feminist geography and medical anthropological theories of health and place, this chapter offers two main contributions. First, it reveals how place is simultaneously held in bodies and reconstituted through memory. Second, it suggests that by pushing out the boundaries of time that separate past from present, it becomes possible to understand that people's experiences of childhood, motherhood, illness and death are not only temporal but also fundamentally, spatial.

6.2 Space and the Place of Memory

The value of thinking about health, illness and death through the lens of memory and space builds on legacies of research in political science, medical anthropology and feminist geography. This section outlines these conceptual framings of space, place, time and memory, and it goes on to integrate and extend these concepts in the subsequent discussion. In this chapter, I conceive space as simultaneously real and contested, and I use the concept of topology, as articulated by Serres and Latour (1995), to capture the construction and fluidity of space. The concept of topology can be traced even further back in time, to 1736, when the Greek-Latin term analysis situs—'the picking apart of a place'—was used by both biologists and mathematicians to map the dimensions of the body and its organs. In a similar vein, Mol and Law (1994) conducted ethnographic research on the management of anaemia by medical doctors. Through this research, they captured their notion of fluid space—or topologies—using blood as a metaphor. They suggest that the difficulty doctors faced in treating anaemia lies in the nature of blood: that, like anaemia itself, it is hard to 'pin down'. In this chapter, I use the concept of topology to indicate the conjunction of shifting spaces and memories and I explore how these topologies are embodied, with memories of illness and health also sometimes hard to 'pin down'.

Like space, I conceive memory as fluid and constructed. To capture this fluidity, I draw on the concept of anamnesis, first offered by Socrates in Plato's *Meno*. Historically, anamnesis was used to reflect iterations of knowledge or the ritual repetition of remembrance. More recently, anamnesis has been described as

> [R]emembrance or reminiscence, the collection and re-collection of what has been lost, forgotten, or effaced. It is therefore a matter of the very old, of what has made us who we are. But anamnesis is also a work that transforms its subject, always producing something new. To recollect the old, to produce the new: that is the task of anamnesis. (Harman 2009: n.p)

The task of anamnesis thus implies a constant remaking of the present through memory. Its contemporary definition indicates how, as a concept, anamnesis draws medical histories and narratives into the present through memory or processes of recollection. In this chapter, anamnesis is explored through a composite collection of narratives linked to women's memories as they (re)constructed their present through narrating their past. Medical anthropological approaches to illness narratives (Kleinman 1989; El Refaie 2019; Egerod et al. 2011) and 'therapeutic narratives' (Mattingly 1998; Lesley 2020; Apud and Romaní 2020) similarly reflect the value of listening to people's memories in their accounts of illness and treatment. In his groundbreaking work, Arthur Kleinman (1989), for example, emphasised the importance of understanding how local social systems inform how bodies and bodily processes are perceived and remembered. In more recent research on memory and HIV in South Africa, anthropologists have similarly suggested that memory works through narrative processes of recollection to mediate the space between people's embodied experience of illness and medicine and the socio-spatial and temporal networks in which they are embedded (Altınay et al. 2019; Cherasia 2020; Colvin 2018).

The memories explored in the findings below centre around women's recollections of embodied precarity linked to HIV and AIDS therapies. I use the term 'precarity' to denote multiple axes of socio-economic inequality that intersect with gender, race, class and age and to discuss how this precarity comes to be embodied by the women I came to know during my fieldwork (Butler 2009; Mills 2017). In doing so, I suggest that the politics of life, coined by Rose (2006) and extended by Fassin (2009), Marsland and Prince (2012), and Dziuban and Sekuler (2021), is not only a question of technologies through which governmentality operates but that it is also a process through which inequalities are (re)produced, embodied and remembered.

6.3 Methods

This article is based on multi-sited ethnography conducted in the first two decades of the twenty-first century. It focuses on ethnographic research conducted from 2010 to 2023 that traced a dynamic network of actors (activists, policy makers, health care systems, pharmaceutical companies) and actants (viruses and medicines) that shaped South African women's access to, and embodiment of, HIV treatment. This fieldwork included ethnographic research with a core group of women who lived in a semi-formal housing area called Khayelitsha in the Cape Town Metropole. This group of women had played a central role in a large-scale social movement, spearheaded by TAC, that challenged the South African government to provide treatment to prevent mother-to-child transmission of

HIV and highly active antiretroviral therapy (ARVs) for the almost five million South Africans who were HIV positive and who would die without access to ARVs (Simelela et al. 2015). The struggle for these medicines took place broadly from 1999 to 2009. Since then, the struggle for ARVs has changed shape, but it has not ended (Kaplan et al. 2017; Osler et al. 2018).

The findings drawn from my work with this core group of activists living in Khayelitsha corroborate the overall findings of the full ethnography that included: 20 key informant interviews with policy actors; 40 narrative life history interviews with men and women on antiretroviral treatment; participant photography and film; and body and journey mapping. The findings discussed in this article centre on field notes generated through participant observation, alongside the photographs and films that were created by the core group of women I worked with. The core group of women all lived in Khayelitsha, were between the ages of 30 and 50 years old and had all worked with TAC in various capacities in the course of the decade-long struggle for ARVs.

Ethics permission for this study was formally obtained through the University of Sussex, through consent forms with each of the study participants, and through ongoing dialogue throughout the course of my research—beyond fieldwork—with the participants to discuss how they would like to be represented, which stories should be shared most boldly and which stories should not be shared at all. The accounts in this article reflect the first type of story.

6.4 Memory, Topologies and Embodiment

The memories of the women with whom I conducted this research shifted back and forth across time in ways that challenge any sense of narrative or teleological linearity. However, for the purpose of clarity, I articulate three pertinent 'topologies' in which these memories were located. The first section traces women's narratives back to the early years of their lives in the Eastern Cape Province. The second section focuses on the socio-spatial construction and performance of gender through a rite of passage that is closely tied to the space—the mountains and 'bush'—of the Eastern Cape. Shifting from the first section that looks at starting life and the second section that explores life transitions, the final section explores women's memories of navigating different healing practices and health resources in the

Eastern and Western Cape provinces in order to sustain their lives and the lives of their children.

6.5 Starting Life: Remembering the Romance and Risk of the Eastern Cape

The women I worked with painted the picture of their past, of their childhood home in the Eastern Cape, with narratives that layered over each other; the layers accrued over time, revealing shifting imaginaries of 'home' as simultaneously beloved and as other. This 'other' was not simply of 'another' place that was reconstructed through memory in order to journey back to the women's previous lives, to places that had made them who they are, that had brought HIV into their bodies and ultimately precipitated their move away from home to Khayelitsha. 'Home' was also an 'other' place held in place by the tension of two narrative strands, one of romance and the other of risk. As anthropologists researching the nature of 'home' have similarly found in their work on migration (Rapport and Dawson 2021) and COVID-19 (Roth et al. 2021), for example, these women's conceptions of 'home' existed in relation to and because of each other, and it was through their juxtaposition that these strands became each other's 'other'.

All of the women I worked with had grown up in the Eastern Cape, and it was here that they believed they had contracted HIV. A predominantly rural part of the country, under-equipped and over-burdened health centres were dotted across the province, and for many women, they offered little hope for health (Coovadia et al. 2009; Vale et al. 2017; Hodes et al. 2017; Gittings et al. 2022). At the turn of the twentieth century, when HIV treatment was first provided through the MSF trial in Khayelitsha (Anderson 2018), it was this tightly circumscribed space in the Western Cape that offered any form of hope for a long life with HIV. However, joining this trial required having a home address in Khayelitsha, and it entailed moving from 'home' in the Eastern Cape.

Miriam, a 36-year-old woman who had been one of the first people to start ARVs on the MSF trial, encapsulated the tension of these two 'homes'. One day, when we were leaving the Site B clinic in Khayelitsha after Miriam's bi-monthly ARV check-up, she explained, "Cape Town's my home because it gave life to my child... I don't even want to tell you how small she was when we got here. But I want to die in the Eastern

Cape because it is the home of my ancestors". The home she describes as being the place of her ancestors is in the Eastern Cape. Miriam had grown up with her mother and two younger brothers in a single round room circumscribed by mud walls and covered by a thatch roof that sheltered them from rain but not from the extreme heat and cold of the shifting seasons. Here, Miriam's family did not have running water or electricity, and she and her mother spent two hours each day walking along the contour path that wound along the hills between their blue-painted home and the nearest river: their sole source of water.

Her mother was chronically ill, and their household's only source of income was her mother's disability grant; occasionally, when they ran out of money, their neighbours would share the few vegetables that they could spare. Miriam said that this (somewhat strained) benevolence ended when their neighbours learnt that her mother had had a relationship with a married man living in the adjacent village; this man was the father of Miriam's two brothers. Like Miriam's own father, he did not provide any form of support to Miriam's mother. This, she explained, was "[Because] men think it's fine. They just want women... They don't care about the children".

Miriam has three photographs that sit on her dressing table in Khayelitsha. These photographs speak to pertinent memories and people in her life. There are two small photographs of her two children graduating from primary school, and a larger photograph, in the centre, where Miriam's 17-year-old self stands in front of her high school and looks directly at the camera. At school, she had dreamt of becoming a teacher but was forced—by her uncle—to leave 3 months before graduating to care for her mother, who had become slowly, irrevocably, incapacitated—poisoned by the wife of the man who had fathered Miriam's brothers. When Miriam's dreamt possibility of becoming a teacher was no longer a potential reality, Miriam 'made do' in De Certeau's (1984) terms by navigating the imperative of taking care of her mother with very few resources as strategically as she could. In part, her decision to enter a sexual relationship with Luyokiso, her first partner, was prompted by Miriam's feeling that "he was the only one caring for me". Without knowledge about HIV or information about sex, more generally, her relationship with Luyokiso was characterised by painful and unprotected sex. Miriam said that she contracted HIV from Luyokiso because a few months after their relationship ended, he had become seriously ill and subsequently died; she believed that he died of AIDS.

Following her mother's death, at the age of 17, Miriam became the head of their household, caring for Nena, her newborn and extremely ill daughter, and her two brothers. Without any financial support (her household could no longer draw on their mother's disability grant), she and her brothers struggled to eat as her child battled to live in the clinic; at a loss, she chose to move with her daughter to Khayelitsha, in the Western Cape, in order to access ARVs.

Miriam's memories of the Eastern Cape as 'other' shifted across the course of my fieldwork, suggesting that these narratives were not rooted in space, as Haraway (1988) suggests, but instead were fluid and co-constructed with space and time. For example, when speaking against Khayelitsha's pollution, its poor sanitation and her struggle with living on the cusp of poverty as her household's sole income earner, Miriam would move to reminisce about her life in the Eastern Cape. She drew pictures in her diary and through our conversations of the lush green valleys and supportive neighbours. Yet, these nostalgic narratives of 'home' sifted under the surface when remembering the social expectations that, as a young woman, she was expected to shoulder the care of her family, and when she told me about the under-resourced clinics and their failure to care for her mother and her daughter in the face of their unyielding illnesses.

Alongside memories linked to the start and end of life in the 'home of the ancestors', the women who—like Miriam—had worked as activists with TAC also described how life in the Eastern Cape became increasingly untenable as they entered adulthood. They spoke of home as a place of risk where gender inequality, poverty and unemployment, and poor health care and education coalesced into multiple forms of precarity, including contracting HIV and transmitting the virus to their babies. Further, it seemed that the shifting memories not only generated the simultaneous romanticisation and othering of 'home' in the Eastern Cape, but that these memories shifted in relation to the women's dynamic relationship to their current home and life in the adjacent Western Cape Province. The following section explores this dynamic with a particular focus on memory and the socio-spatial generation of gender through rites of passage.

6.6 Marking Life: Memory and the Socio-spatial Generation of Gender

The gendered expectations of care that so powerfully shaped Miriam's life were, according to the women I worked with, inculcated through rites of passage that took place in the space of the Eastern Cape. The Eastern Cape was recollected by the research participants as the socio-spatial repository of *isiXhosa* cultural knowledge. This knowledge was, as articulated below, held in memories and in bodies, transmitted across generations through rites of passage that include circumcision, marriage ceremonies and funerals. This section focuses on male circumcision in particular and explores the tension between, on the one hand, the women's assertion of the importance of affirming ties to family and ancestral homes and, on the other hand, their struggle with the implicit and, at times, explicit construction of gender roles through these same practices that reinforce kinship ties. The purpose of this sub-section is not to reflect on the larger social and policy dynamics linked to circumcision. Instead, it points to the relationship between the space of the Eastern Cape, the timing of this rite of passage and specific local cultural practices linked to circumcision.

Each year, in December, many of the women in my research were preparing to journey east along the N2 highway—the main artery connecting the Western and Eastern Cape Provinces—to celebrate Christmas with their families. December is also a time of year marked by the flow of boys on the cusp of manhood as they travel to the Eastern Cape to undergo traditional male circumcision 'in the bush' (a reference to the oblique space in which this practice, shrouded in mystery for women, takes place). In the first year that we knew each other, Miriam carefully saved up the large amount of money required to send her 23-year-old brother, Masiphiwe, to be circumcised. At this time, Yvonne also travelled to her partner's homestead in the Eastern Cape to celebrate his brother's return 'from the bush'. Prior to travelling home, Yvonne spent weeks wondering whether or not to join her partner in celebrating his brother's return from 'the bush'. She was concerned that she would be corralled into performing the role of 'wife' and given onerous responsibilities. In the excerpt below, Yvonne reflects on the way women are expected to perform deference to men when they become 'wives':

> Although we're not married, they still expect me to be the wife. It's like a compliment, almost. They want to treat me like a daughter... But also, they want me to behave like a wife. To be silent; to take care of their son; to only be with other [married] women.

Yvonne did make the trip, and when she came back from the Eastern Cape, she spoke of her relief in returning to the life that she had built in Khayelitsha with her mother and her son, a life where she was not primarily identified as a partner or wife.

In their accounts of this rite of passage, Yvonne and Miriam moved between, on the one hand, remembering the place of the Eastern Cape romantically as the socio-spatial repository of important cultural knowledge that was becoming eroded through linked processes of urbanisation and modernisation in peri-urban areas like Khayelitsha. On the other hand, they also recalled how the Eastern Cape functioned as the place where, because of these cultural practices, men were compelled to perform particular kinds of masculinities that, in turn, correlated with expectations for how women should defer to the authority of men in social and sexual relationships.

Expressing a similar ambivalence towards circumcision, Zama said that she would make sure her 6-year-old son, Lwazi, was circumcised because it was vital for his entry into adulthood, but that she would ensure that in the intervening years, he learnt, by watching her live her life, that women were deserving of respect. This rationale underpinned her decision to end her relationship with Lwazi's abusive father; she was concerned that her son would learn, through observing his father's abuse, to disrespect women. She was therefore resigned to the importance of circumcision as a rite of passage while also deeply suspicious about this rite as a tool used by men to transmit discriminatory constructions of gender hierarchies that place men at the pinnacle under the guise of 'tradition'.

6.7 Sustaining Life: The Memory of Illness in the 'Brown Map' of Skin

Most of the women I worked with learned that they were HIV-positive in the late 1990s and early 2000s, at a time when the government failed to provide ARVs (Hodes 2018). As we heard from Miriam above, the location of MSF's ARV trial in Khayelitsha, in the Western Cape Province, was an important aspect of the women's memories of Khayelitsha as a life-giving place in contrast to the Eastern Cape, where most remember contracting HIV and first becoming seriously ill. Like the geographic location of the two provinces themselves, these two spaces (of 'home' in the Eastern Cape and Khayelitsha in the Western Cape) danced along a narrative seesaw, counterpoints to each other: factors that enabled HIV to enter the women's bodies were attributed to topologies of 'home' in the Eastern Cape, and those that had facilitated access to AIDS therapies were attributed to topologies of Khayelitsha. In this final section, we see how these memories of space-time shift depending on the location of the narration.

Zama was preparing to travel back 'home' along the N2 highway to be with her sister's family for Christmas in the Eastern Cape, and we met up for tea before she left. Sitting near her office in a small suburb outside Cape Town, I asked her to tell me more about her home in the Eastern Cape. Although we had known each other for almost a decade, I was not entirely clear about her life outside of the world that we shared in the Western Cape. Zama told me that her 'home' was a place with 'green-smelling air', with grassy valleys and views of green far into the distance; she spoke of the river that she swam in and that she, her mother and sisters would use for their household's cooking and cleaning. I asked her to take some photographs of her time back 'home', and when Zama returned, we sat down to look at them together. After a series of photographs taken at night to mark the stops along the N2 highway, we moved into daylight and a photograph was taken out of the window of the minibus taxi she was travelling on with her son and a friend's child of the same age. The photograph was of a green open space dotted with trees against a sloping hill. "Here is our toilet", she said. The next photograph was of about 100 pastel-painted Reconstruction and Development Programme (RDP) houses:

> Nothing works in these houses. The government wanted to look like they were doing something good for us. But they just built us walls. Like empty shells.

Gloria lived in one of these pastel RDP houses with her children and her partner, and it was here that Zama was based for Christmas. Zama said that she used a bucket at night-time, instead of leaving the safety of their home, because she had heard that women had recently been raped when they had gone out at night to the open place that functioned as the community's toilet space. This memory contrasts with her account, prior to her trip, of home as a place of safety.

A few days into her trip, Zama, Gloria and their children travelled to their father's plot up in the valley; a few years previously, her father had sought permission from the village chief to build a home. The home reflects her parents' wish to move from their small shack in Khayelitsha to this village, but the reality of the remote rural location has meant that Zama's father was forced to stop the construction. The house still stood on the land, half built, with mud and grass meshed into the trees that had been stripped and tied together to form walls. Tilled earth, also ringed by a fence of trimmed tree trunks, was a visible reminder of another memory: in 2003, Zama's brother, Sihle, had become frustrated with his life in Khayelitsha and decided to return to his father's land in order to try to make this home his own. Sihle was frustrated, as Zama recounted, with "The concrete buildings everywhere and the bad air", and so he sought a referral letter from the MSF clinic, where he received his ARVs, to relocate. Sihle needed to travel to Lusikisiki each month to get his ARVs: it was the only place, aside from Khayelitsha, that provided ARVs through MSF at that time. Unable to afford the cost of the return taxi journey to Lusikisiki from his home high up in the mountains, about three hours away, Sihle stopped taking ARVs. He became very sick very quickly in the course of a month and, financial cost aside, was too frail to attempt the journey to the clinic to access his ARVs.

Sihle's father travelled back to their home in the Eastern Cape to bring Sihle to Khayelitsha. Also extremely frail, he carried Sihle on his back and then in a wheelbarrow along winding routes down the mountain over almost impassable mud roads. When they reached the larger tar road, they were able to get into a minibus taxi and start the slow, long journey back along the N2 highway to their other home in Khayelitsha.

As Zama recounted this longer history, held in the image of her family's half-built home, she also started to tell me of her own journey. We travelled between her memories of Khayelitsha and her family's home, the Eastern Cape, as her memories of first becoming ill overlaid each other. When Zama first became very seriously ill in 1999, she sought treatment with an *isangoma* (traditional healer). Her illness was embodied as drastic weight loss, chronic joint pain, difficulty in breathing and a painful skin condition. The *isangoma* confirmed her suspicion of witchcraft, saying that she had been bewitched to be a snake because her neighbours were jealous of her education. At the time Zama became ill, she had just completed training to be a security guard. Her illness had made it difficult to work, and she had returned, like many of the women I worked with, to the Eastern Cape to be cared for by her extended family.

The recollection of witchcraft made sense to Zama. Alongside this sense-making, which I turn to below, Zama was latently aware that she may be HIV-positive—an aetiology that also made a degree of sense, but that was significantly more frightening in the absence of ARVs and in the presence of vicious stigma borne through misinformation. This shifting process of sense-making points to multiple intersecting conceptions of illness and the sedimentation of memories that accompany this sense-making of bodies that become frail in the search for healing.

The quieter narrative of HIV was layered into her belief that she had been bewitched, for two reasons: one, because Sihle, whom we met earlier, had experienced a similar set of illnesses, and had tested HIV-positive; two, because she had been told by the sister of a previous partner, that he was HIV-positive. Perhaps, rather than distinguishing between the two strands of memories, as one might if trying to make sense of Zama's sense-making from the outside, we can see that, for Zama, these strands are layered into each other through anamnesis. There were times, for example, when Zama spoke to me of being bewitched to be HIV-positive.

In this respect, understanding the relationship between memory and place might extend the historical medical anthropological approach to illness narratives (cf. Kleinman 1989; Kleinman and Kleinman 1994) because it moves away from linear narrative accounts to recognising how we constantly reconstitute ourselves through shifting memories of place, where the things that have made us who we are, that have in some cases made us ill, also shift over time and space and come to be layered into each other. Further, the critique of representationalism held in Haraway's (1991) account of material-semiotics suggests value in moving beyond binaries in which Zama's account of illness is either material (linked to the presence of the virus in her body) or semiotic (linked to witchdoctors that make the skies fight and engender illness). Zama's account suggests, instead, that her experience of embodied illness is both material *and* semiotic, shifting and settling over time and in different spaces.

Through an iterative sedimentation of memory, Zama related the multiple beliefs she held to make sense of her body's illness. At the time she became ill, ARVs were not available; biomedical treatment was not a viable option. Traditional healing, on the other hand, made sense for Zama at this time and in the space of the Eastern Cape because it was a healing strategy that she understood and that conferred a degree of control to her in a situation that had otherwise felt utterly perplexing.

Talking about this time retrospectively, Zama also recounted her initial engagement with TAC in 2001, having travelled back to Khayelitsha at her brother Sihle's insistence to test for HIV. It was through MSF that she first accessed ARVs, and through TAC that she learnt about the science of HIV. Looking back in time to her younger self, she reasoned that, in fact, the witch doctors were not responsible for her illness. In the course of 'sense-making' through anamnesis, Zama made sense of her decision to see an *isangoma* because she wanted to locate the responsibility for her illness with social ill will between herself and her neighbours, thus also affirming her relative success rather than foregrounding her dismay at her shedding skin and inexplicably ill body. Therefore, at that space-time, the narrative of bewitchment was most salient because the narrative of HIV was far more daunting and, at that time and in that place, without ARVs, impossible to heal. Zama's memories, told through as a form of illness narrative, suggest that there is not necessarily a clear distinction between biomedical care and traditional healing in South Africa. Instead, a plurality of health care approaches exist alongside each other, sometimes moving into and reinforcing each other at different junctures of space-time (Shuster et al. 2009; Peltzer et al. 2008; Wreford 2008; Ordóñez 2021; Zuma et al. 2017; Galvin et al. 2023).

The memory of this time in her life is embodied in the present, still visible as light marks on Zama's skin. The *isangoma's* explanation for Zama's illness, namely that she had been bewitched to be a snake, resonated because of the condition of her skin at that time, a condition that had made parts of her skin go grey and dark in colour against the lighter brown of her skin. Almost absentmindedly touching my wrist as we were talking, Zama pulled her long sleeves up over her forearm and then pointed to the trousers covering her legs; over a decade later, the effect of illness was still evident in the tiny dark circles that moved up and down her skin, the skin she describes as a 'brown map'. Looking back to the time when she was very sick, as told through the story of this 'brown map', Zama said that her skin was akin to that of a snake: hard imbrications of flaky skin that reminded her of the "supposed to be soft but really rough skin" that snakes shed as they grow.

Her memory of becoming very seriously ill also connects to the space of home at a time when she initially sought treatment for being bewitched with an *isangoma*; she describes the space of her home as one where HIV was unknown, and where traditional health practitioners were the primary providers of care to ill people. This space connects with the time that Zama became ill, the dearth of information around HIV prevention and the complete absence of treatment in South Africa's public health system in 1999. Zama's description of her skin as a 'brown map' iterates the intersection of space and time, a space-time that her body bears witness to through the fine circles that, although lighter, still lie on her skin. This form of embodied anamnesis, retold through layered illness narratives and visually held in her skin, not only draws time and space together, but also indicates how the past is held in the present in Zama's body.

6.8 Conclusion

In engaging with topology through the lens of social theory, Mol and Law (1994) argue that the social does not exist in a single space, but rather that it is performed in several kinds of space. These different kinds of space are described as 'fluid' where neither boundaries nor relations mark the difference between one place and another. "Instead, sometimes boundaries come and go, allow leakage or disappear altogether, while relations transform themselves... Sometimes, then, social space behaves like a *fluid*" (1994: 643). The way in which the women I worked with remembered HIV and ARVs entering their lives and becoming animated in their bodies was a narrative (re)construction that, like blood and networks, constantly shifted, thus rendering space and time fluid, remade through memory.

By exploring memories across three salient times—starting life, life transitions and sustaining life—this chapter emphasises fluidity and partiality in the unending task of sense-making through the process of narrative recollection. Perhaps it is precisely this dynamic of narrative that lies at the heart of understanding HIV and memory, as people dialogue with their own recollections of where they have come from to (re)construct who and where they are. The memories that are woven into the women's accounts in this chapter are salient in both their form and their substance.

In their form, the memories extend from verbal recollection and reconstructions and include things that were unspoken. Stories of past and present are held in the photographs of Miriam's children in their school in Khayelitsha next to the photograph of Miriam at 17 in front of her school in the Eastern Cape; in diary entries containing words and drawings of stories that were not, could not be, spoken about; in the partially built wood-and-sand home in the Eastern Cape that belongs to Zama's father, a legacy of a former life and potential for another way of living that Zama longs for when she is in Khayelitsha, and also derides when visiting this site 'back home'. In this article, therefore, memories reflect a collection of stories that are simultaneously material and semiotic, that shift back and forth between past and present.

In their substance, the memories were co-constructed with space and time and held in the bodies of women. For example, women's accounts of the pathways that brought HIV into their bodies imply an 'othering' of their childhood homes in the Eastern Cape as places that rendered their bodies precarious. However, when the women spoke of their anxiety about poverty in Khayelitsha, for example, the romance of the Eastern Cape's green valleys and safe villages became salient. As such, the narrative threads of anamnesis are socio-spatial and partial, depending on the kinds of memories that are invoked in different places and across different times. These memories articulate with space-time, suggesting that where people are located in these spatialities shapes how their partial perspectives and memories unfold. Therefore, this article suggests that memories generated through narrative (re)construction are spatialised and, further, it demonstrates that situated knowledge, in contrast with Haraway's (2020) conceptualisation, is not static but constantly (re)negotiated through the dynamism of anamnesis in which embodied memories of starting, marking, and sustaining life shift and change across space and time.

I conclude this article just after returning from fieldwork, where I sat with Zama in Cape Town's summer sunshine. She was about to travel across to the Eastern Cape with her 5-year-old son; her oldest son, Lwazi, had started his initiation, and she would travel across to be with him and to celebrate his transition into manhood when he returned from 'the bush' in early January 2024. In contrast to her sense of wariness about this pivotal rite of passage over 10 years ago, now she had witnessed him grow into a young man who would soon train to be a nurse and of whom she was enormously proud. I recollected the conversation we had had when Lwazi was 6, and Zama pointed out that my child, also 6, will grow in ways I cannot begin to imagine. Bringing my present-day experience of parenthood into dialogue with her own journey of navigating illness, health and parenting, I learnt again from her about the power of imagination and the importance of engaging the unexpected as we move into the future.

References

Altınay, Ayşe Gül, María José Contreras, Marianne Hirsch, Jean Howard, Banu Karaca, and Alisa Solomon. 2019. *Women Mobilizing Memory*. New York: Columbia University Press.

Anderson, Jessica L. 2018. Global humanitarian Organizations and African goals: The Case of Médecins Sans Frontières in South Africa. In *African Foreign Policies in International Institutions*, ed. Jason Warner and Timothy M. Shaw, 229–244. New York: Springer.

Apud, Ismael, and Oriol Romaní. 2020. Medical Anthropology and Symbolic Cure: From the Placebo to Cultures of Meaningful Healing. *Anthropology & Medicine* 27 (2): 160–175.

Biehl, João. 2007. *Will to Live: AIDS Therapies and the Politics of Survival*. Princeton: Princeton University Press.

———. 2013. Ethnography in the Way of Theory. *Cultural Anthropology* 28 (4): 573–597.

Biehl, João, and Peter Locke. 2017. *Unfinished: The Anthropology of Becoming*. Durham: Duke University Press.

Butler, Judith. 2009. Performativity, Precarity and Sexual Politics. *Antropólogos Iberoamericanos en Red (AIBR)* 4 (3): 321–336.

Cancelliere, Francesca. 2020. The Politics of Adherence to Antiretroviral Therapy: Between Ancestral Conflicts and Drug Resistance. *DADA Rivista di Antropologia post-globale* 2: 13–41.

Chapman, Rachel R. 2021. Therapeutic borderlands: Austerity, Maternal HIV Treatment, and the ElusiveEend of AIDS in Mozambique. *Medical Anthropology Quarterly* 35 (2): 226–245.

Cherasia, Spencer P. 2020. Affordances, Remediation, and Digital Mourning: A Comparative Case Study of Two AIDS Memorials. *Memory Studies*. https://doi.org/10.1177/1750698019894686.

Colvin, Christopher J. 2018. *Traumatic Storytelling and Memory in Post-Apartheid South Africa: Performing Signs of Injury*. London: Routledge.

Coovadia, Hoosen, Rachel Jewkes, Peter Barron, David Sanders, and Diane McIntyre. 2009. The Health and Health System of South Africa: Historical Roots of Current Public Health Challenges. *The Lancet* 374 (9692): 817–834.

Copeland, Toni. 2018. To Keep This Disease from Killing You: Cultural Competence, Consonance, and Health Among HIV-Positive Women in Kenya. *Medical Anthropology Quarterly* 32 (2): 272–292.

De Certeau, M. 1984. *The Practice of Everyday Life*. Berkeley: University of California Press.

Dziuban, Agata, and Todd Sekuler. 2021. The Temporal Regimes of HIV/AIDS Activism in Europe: Chrono-Citizenship, Biomedicine and Its Others. *Critical Public Health* 31 (1): 5–16.

Egerod, Ingrid, Doris Christensen, Katherine Hvid Schwartz-Nielsen, and Anne Sophie Ågård. 2011. Constructing the Illness Narrative: A Grounded Theory Exploring Patients' and Relatives' Use of Intensive Care Diaries. *Critical Care Medicine* 39 (8): 1922–1928.

El Refaie, Elisabeth. 2019. *Visual Metaphor and Embodiment in Graphic Illness Narratives*. New York: Oxford University Press.

Fassin, Didier. 2009. Another Politics of Life Is Possible. *Theory, Culture & Society* 26 (5): 44–60.

Galvin, Michael, Lesley Chiwaye, and Aneesa Moolla. 2023. Religious and Medical Pluralism Among Traditional Healers in Johannesburg, South Africa. *Journal of Religion and Health* 63 (2): 907–923.

Gittings, Lesley, Christopher J. Colvin, and Rebecca Hodes. 2022. Blood and Blood: Anti-retroviral Therapy, Masculinity, and Redemption among Adolescent Boys in the Eastern Cape Province of South Africa. *Medical Anthropology Quarterly* 36 (3): 367–390.

Haraway, D. 1988. Situated knowledges: The Science Question in Feminism and the Privilege of Partial Perspective. *Feminist Studies* 14 (3): 575–599.

Haraway, D.J. 1991. *Simians, Cyborgs and Women: The Reinvention of Nature*. London: Free Association.

Haraway, Donna. 2020. Situated Knowledges: The Science Question in Feminism and the Privilege of Partial Perspective. In *Feminist Theory Reader*, ed. Carole McCann, Seung-kyung Kim, and Emek Ergun, 303–310. New York: Routledge.

Harman, G. 2009. *Prince of Networks: Bruno LaTour and Metaphysics*. Melbourne: Re.Press.

Hodes, Rebecca. 2018. HIV/AIDS in South Africa. In *Oxford Research Encyclopedia of African History*, ed. T. Spear. Oxford: Oxford University Press.

Hodes, R., I. Price, N. Bungane, E. Toska, and L. Cluver. 2017. How Front-Line Healthcare Workers Respond to Stock-Outs of Essential Medicines in the Eastern Cape Province of South Africa. *South African Medical Journal* 107 (9): 738–740.

Johnson, Leigh F., and Rob E. Dorrington. 2023. Modelling the Impact of HIV in South Africa's Provinces: 2023 Update. In *Centre for Infectious Disease Epidemiology and Research Working Paper*. Cape Town: Centre for Infectious Disease Epidemiology and Research.

Kalofonos, Ippolytos Andreas. 2008. *"All I Eat is ARVs": Living with HIV/AIDS at the Dawn of the Treatment Era in*. Central Mozambique: ProQuest.

Kaplan, Samantha R., Christa Oosthuizen, Kathryn Stinson, Francesca Little, Jonathan Euvrard, Michael Schomaker, Meg Osler, Katherine Hilderbrand, Andrew Boulle, and Graeme Meintjes. 2017. Contemporary disengagement from Antiretroviral Therapy in Khayelitsha, South Africa: A Cohort Study. *PLoS Medicine* 14 (11): e1002407.

Kleinman, A. 1989. *The Illness Narratives: Suffering, Healing, and The Human Condition*. New York, Basic Books.

Kleinman, Arthur, and Joan Kleinman. 1994. How Bodies Remember: Social Memory and Bodily Experience of Criticism, Resistance, and Delegitimation Following China's Cultural Revolution. *New Literary History* 25 (3): 707–723.

Larkan, Fiona. 2004. Narratives and Silences in Discussions of AIDS/HIV Amongst Young People in Mpumalanga, South Africa. *Irish Journal of Anthropology* 7.

Larkan, Fiona, B. Van Wyk, P. Stevens, and A.J. Saris. 2015. Between the Clinic and the Community: Temporality and Patterns of ART Adherence in the Western Cape Province, South Africa. *African Sociological Review/Revue Africaine de Sociologie* 19 (2): 26–52.

Lesley, Elena. 2020. Immaterial Alliances: Constructions of Self-Other Relations and Conceptions of Belonging in the Therapeutic Narratives of Muslim and Buddhist Cambodians. *Ethos* 48 (3): 379–399.

Marsland, Rebecca. 2012. (Bio)Sociality and HIV in Tanzania: Finding a Living to Support a Life. *Medical Anthropology Quarterly* 26 (4): 470–485. https://doi.org/10.1111/maq.12002.

Marsland, Rebecca, and Ruth Prince. 2012. What is Life Worth? Exploring Biomedical Interventions, Survival, and the Politics of Life. *Medical Anthropology Quarterly* 26 (4): 453–469. https://doi.org/10.1111/maq.12001.

Mattes, Dominik. 2019. *Fierce Medicines, Fragile Socialities: Grounding Global HIV Treatment in Tanzania*. Vol. 18. New York: Berghahn Books.

Mattingly, C. 1998. *Healing Dramas and Clinical Plots: The Narrative Structure of Experience*. Vol. 7. Cambridge: Cambridge University Press.

Mills, Elizabeth. 2017. Biopolitical Precarity in the Permeable Body: The Social Lives of People, Viruses and Their Medicines. *Critical Public Health* 27 (3): 350–361.

Mol, A., and J. Law. 1994. Regions, Networks and Fluids: Anaemia and Social Topology. *Social Studies of Science* 24 (4): 641–671.

Musyoki, Helgar, Parinita Bhattacharjee, Keith Sabin, Ed Ngoksin, Tisha Wheeler, and Gina Dallabetta. 2021. A Decade and Beyond: Learnings from HIV Programming with Underserved and Marginalized Key Populations in Kenya. *Journal of the International AIDS Society* 24: e25729.

Nance, Nerissa, Prosper Pendo, Joseph Masanja, David Paul Ngilangwa, Karen Webb, Rita Noronha, and Sandra I. McCoy. 2017. Short-Term Effectiveness of a Community Health Worker Intervention for HIV-Infected Pregnant Women in Tanzania to Improve Treatment Adherence and Retention in Care: A Cluster-Randomized Trial. *PLoS One* 12 (8): e0181919.

Ordóñez, Claudia E. 2021. Coordination of Medical Pluralism in Public HIV Health Care in South Africa. In *Living with HIV in Post-crisis Times: Beyond the Endgame*, ed. David A.B. Murray, 81. Lanham: Lexington Books.
Osler, Meg, Katherine Hilderbrand, Eric Goemaere, Nathan Ford, Mariette Smith, Graeme Meintjes, James Kruger, Nelesh P. Govender, and Andrew Boulle. 2018. The Continuing Burden of Advanced HIV Disease over 10 Years of Increasing Antiretroviral Therapy Coverage in South Africa. *Clinical Infectious Diseases* 66 (suppl_2): S118–S125.
Peltzer, Karl, Natalie F. Preez, Shandir Ramlagan, and Henry Fomundam. 2008. Use of Traditional Complementary and Alternative Medicine for HIV Patients in KwaZulu-Natal, South Africa. *BMC public Health* 8 (1): 255.
Pillay-van Wyk, V., W. Msemburi, R.E. Dorrington, R. Laubscher, Pamela Groenewald, and Debbie Bradshaw. 2019. HIV/AIDS Mortality Trends Pre and Post ART for 1997-2012 in South Africa—Have We Turned the Tide? *South African Medical Journal* 109 (11b): 41–44.
Prince, Ruth. 2012. HIV and the Moral Economy of Survival in an East African City. *Medical Anthropology Quarterly* 26 (4): 534–556. https://doi.org/10.1111/maq.12006.
Rapport, Nigel, and Andrew Dawson. 2021. Home and Movement: A Polemic. In *Migrants of Identity*, ed. Andrew Dawson and Nigel Rapport, 19–38. London: Routledge.
Rose, Nikolas. 2006. *The Politics of Life Itself: Biomedicine, Power and Subjectivity in the Twenty-First Century*. Princeton: Princeton University Press.
Roth, Adam, Niroshnee Ranjan, Grace King, Shamim Homayun, Rebecca Hendershott, and Simone Dennis. 2021. Zooming in on COVID: The intimacies of Screens, Homes and Learning Hierarchies. *Anthropology in Action* 28 (1): 67–72.
Serres, Michel, and Bruno Latour. 1995. *Conversations on Science, Culture, and Time*. Ann Arbor: University of Michigan Press.
Shuster, Justin M., Claire E. Sterk, Paula M. Frew, and Carlos Del Rio. 2009. The Cultural and Community-Level Acceptance of Antiretroviral Therapy (ART) Among Traditional Healers in Eastern Cape, South Africa. *Journal of Community Health* 34 (1): 16–22.
Simelela, Nono, W.D. Francois Venter, Yogan Pillay, and Peter Barron. 2015. A Political and Social History of HIV in South Africa. *Current HIV/AIDS Reports* 12 (2): 256–261.
Vale, Beth, Rebecca Hodes, and Lucie Cluver. 2017. Negotiations of Blame and Care Among HIV-Positive Mothers and Daughters in South Africa's Eastern Cape. *Medical Anthropology Quarterly* 31 (4): 519–536.
Wilson, Herieth Ismael, and Herry Mapesi. 2020. Rollout of Dolutegravir-Based Antiretroviral Therapy in Sub-Saharan Africa and Its Public Health Implications. *The Pan African Medical Journal* 37.

Wreford, Jo Thobeka. 2008. *Working with Spirit: Experiencing Izangoma Healing in Contemporary South Africa*. New York: Berghahn Books.

Young, Ingrid, Mark Davis, Paul Flowers, and Lisa M. McDaid. 2019. Navigating HIV Citizenship: Identities, Risks and Biological Citizenship in the Treatment as Prevention Era. *Health, Risk & Society* 21 (1–2): 1–16.

Zuma, Thembelihle, Daniel Wight, Tamsen Rochat, and Mosa Moshabela. 2017. Traditional Health Practitioners' Management of HIV/AIDS in Rural South Africa in the Era of Widespread Antiretroviral Therapy. *Global Health Action* 10 (1): 1352210.

CHAPTER 7

Mothering with HIV

Denise Proudfoot and Ellie Marley

7.1 Introduction

Women account for nearly over half of all new HIV diagnoses around the world (UNAIDS 2022). Nevertheless, since early in the HIV pandemic, the lives/experiences of women/mothers living with HIV have received little attention. Importantly, there has been a lack of research on the highly gendered implications of an HIV diagnosis (Tariq and Kasadha 2022). To date, much HIV research with women has tended to focus on transmission, prevention and treatment phenomena (Logan-Kennedy et al. 2014), which perceives women with children through a narrow set of 'motherhood' discourses and practices and, therefore, much less is known about their lives. The continued lack of research about women and mothers living with HIV impacts their care and support needs (Tariq and Kasadha 2022). Even now, in the fifth decade of this pandemic, due to the wide availability of effective treatments, many further complexities relating to having and rearing children when HIV positive are often neglected. Central to this chapter will be a discussion of the maternal HIV

D. Proudfoot (✉) • E. Marley
Dublin City University, Dublin, Ireland
e-mail: denise.proudfoot@dcu.ie

A. Castillo Villanueva, A. Bollas (eds.), *HIV/AIDS in Memory, Culture and Society*, Palgrave Studies in Science and Popular Culture, https://doi.org/10.1007/978-3-031-59699-5_7

experience, which draws on qualitative research interviews with support from historical, cultural and sociological contexts as they relate to HIV. The study, which underpins the chapter discussion, was with Irish-based mothers living with HIV (MLHIV) and provides insight into the maternal HIV experience while privileging their individual mothering narratives and giving a voice to these women.

Women living with HIV (WLHIV) are diverse and come from all sections of society, including professionals, students, migrants and women who work in a variety of sectors; some are mothers/grandmothers, mothers who have lost children to HIV/AIDS, and identify as heterosexual, lesbian and/or transgender women. Some have lived with HIV for decades; others are newly diagnosed or born with HIV. Gaining an understanding of the female HIV experience is crucial because HIV affects men and women differently (Walsh et al. 2012), and having children will have a major impact on this experience. For many women, becoming a mother is a natural part of life; however, a health condition like HIV can complicate this process and their mothering experiences and lives overall.

This chapter will discuss the maternal HIV experiences relevant across multiple eras of HIV, spanning from before AZT medication was available to the current U=U era. It will explore and discuss issues relating to Irish-based mothers with reference to research that examined the effects of this diagnosis on mothers. It will also take account of how the changes and advances in HIV treatments from the AZT era to the contemporary HIV picture have affected the maternal HIV experience considering the life-changing impact of this diagnosis and the often highly gendered implications of this condition.

7.2 Issues for Mothers Living with HIV

There has been much criticism of HIV biomedical success since it does not address all the issues HIV raises in people's lives. The emotional and psychological implications of being diagnosed with HIV (Walker 2019) remain for some. Stigma has been widely cited as having detrimental effects on people living with HIV's mental health, including mothers (Nobre et al. 2018; Rice et al. 2018; Sikstrom 2018; Cuca et al. 2017; Hutchinson and Dhairyawan 2017; Sangaramoorthy et al. 2017; Bennett et al. 2016; Brion et al. 2014). Very often, these areas of omission or neglect relate to the gendered and sexualised characteristics of the HIV pandemic, as well as to psychosocial issues. Mothering with HIV takes many forms. The experiences of women becoming mothers or not having children have strongly been shaped by the availability of HAART to prevent vertical transmission. Vertical transmission is the term adopted to describe when HIV is passed onto a foetus or newborn baby during pregnancy, labour, delivery or breastfeeding (WHO 2024).

For WLHIV who want to become mothers post diagnosis, a considerable amount of decision-making is involved (Toupin et al. 2019; Cuca and Dawson Rose 2016). This can include issues around trusting the effectiveness of medication to prevent their babies from being infected with HIV, the worry of stigma and the discomfort of women who feel ashamed of their diagnosis (Toupin et al. 2019; Greene et al. 2015). For these women, their pregnancy experience is highly managed to ensure the prevention of vertical transmission, and the quality of their relationships with healthcare providers is of great importance to that experience (McCarthy et al. 2014). Furthermore, decision-making regarding having children as a woman living with HIV is compounded by the persistent stigmatising discourse that women are vectors, and women who are HIV positive and have children are reckless and irresponsible as they can pass HIV on to their children (Zivi 2005). Negotiating the risk of vertical transmission and the risk of societal stigma of being an HIV-positive mother can often inform the decisions these women face regarding their fertility (Toupin et al. 2019). The experience for women has shifted dramatically over the past 40 years as they are now assured that as long as they are on treatment throughout their pregnancy, vertical transmission can be prevented, although studies have highlighted that this concern remains for many pregnant women with HIV (Toupin et al. 2019; Proudfoot 2014).

In many cultures, women deal with social and cultural expectations about their lives, and this includes becoming mothers. However, for many women who have been diagnosed with HIV, their diagnosis disrupts this journey due to societal stigma. Accordingly, WLHIV's journey towards motherhood must extend beyond a physiological discussion and incorporate societal and cultural issues informing the experiences of WLHIV (Anderson 2012).

For women diagnosed as part of antenatal screening, the impact on their pregnancy experience is multifactorial (Toupin et al. 2019; Proudfoot 2018; Kelly et al. 2012). Women diagnosed with HIV during pregnancy are required to take life-long medication as well as adjust to their diagnosis (Proudfoot 2018). For women who are diagnosed with HIV during their first pregnancy, a biographical disruption in the dual context of HIV and pregnancy can occur (Bury 1982). Biographical disruption refers to a change in the anticipated life that one imagines for oneself due to the onset of a chronic condition (Bury 1982). Some expectant mothers who were diagnosed prior to the advent of HAART were faced with the concern of how long they would live to see their child/children grow up, combined with the fear of possible vertical transmission (Proudfoot 2018). Again, women's experiences are strongly contextualised by the era in which their diagnosis during pregnancy took place. However, research describes how the burden of an HIV diagnosis for women during pregnancy is significant, no matter what stage of the HIV pandemic it occurred (Proudfoot 2018; Kelly et al. 2012).

Mothers who were diagnosed during the early years of the HIV pandemic faced the dilemma of whether they would see their children grow up (Barnes et al. 1997). Today, due to the success of HAART as a medical treatment globally, this is not typically considered a cause for concern because an HIV diagnosis no longer means a premature death. However, due to the persistence of HIV stigma, some mothers believe their HIV diagnosis could affect their children should their HIV-positive status become known, and, furthermore, they also worry about whether to tell their children that they are living with HIV (Proudfoot 2014). Finally, throughout this chapter, we must acknowledge women who were diagnosed with HIV early on in the HIV pandemic and whose journey to motherhood was impeded by an HIV diagnosis, as many women were discouraged from becoming pregnant to avoid vertical transmission of HIV (Desclaux and Cadart 2008).

Another important consideration is that the general visibility of pregnancy and motherhood balanced against the invisibility and often hidden nature of their HIV status (in the era of successful treatment) can pose significant distress for WLHIV. Even in the fifth decade of HIV, it remains a highly stigmatised condition for many. For women, the association between sex and HIV is particularly poignant. When pregnant, women's bodies often become the subject of public discussion, in which societies often feel they are afforded an opinion on women's bodies in terms of what they should and shouldn't do to protect a growing foetus inside them (De-Vitri Smith et al. 2013; Bailey 2001). This extends to the social and medical societal expectations relating to women having children (De-Vitri Smith et al. 2013). Mothering and child-rearing can be heavily critiqued and criticised by society, again, born out of a place of welfare for a child, but it is likely a patriarchal exertion of control over women and their actions in the important role that child-rearing entails. The HIV-positive body has often been the subject of public discussion regarding HIV infectivity and public health, although this sentiment has strongly been tainted with HIV stigma (Persson 2013). The prevalence and persistence of the stigmatising discourse surrounding HIV, in particularly pregnancy and motherhood among women living with HIV, positioned women as vectors of disease who were putting the unborn at risk, or they were even considered reckless for becoming pregnant in the first instance, and as such these factors challenged what it means to be a 'good mother' in the eyes of society. Zivi's (2005) work describes societal views of 'good mothers' as women who embody characteristics such as nurturance and selflessness and 'bad mothers' as women who neglect and put their children in danger, sadly echoing the stigmatising discourse that women and mothers are faced with as 'vectors of disease'. Women who are pregnant and/or mothers and living with HIV can be challenged with keeping HIV invisible to protect their identity as a mother considering such stigma (Toupin et al. 2019; Cuca and Dawson Rose 2016; Zivi 2005) because HIV is still associated with sexual promiscuity in many societies (Carter et al. 2017; Nevedal and Sankar 2016; Davtyan et al. 2016). This can potentially hinder a woman's ability to relate to the norm of the 'good mother', as common maternal ideologies affect both women's HIV and mothering experiences. The unrealistic 'perfect' mother image persists in many contexts, and feminist scholars challenge this concept because they argue that the reality for many women is more complex (O'Reilly 2014). This is especially so for women who 'mother' in challenging circumstances. Contemporary social and cultural discourses of maternity shape the mothering experiences of women living with HIV and gaining an understanding of the maternal HIV experience demonstrates that having children will have a major impact on their lives.

7.3 Women and HIV in Ireland: The Early Years

Many Western societies consider motherhood to be a central pillar and aspiration for women to fulfil their social roles. The current Irish Constitution emphasises that the place of women in society is closely linked to motherhood, and for decades, the Catholic Church affected and controlled Irish family size, women's reproductive health and child-rearing (Hug 1998). The 20 years between the 1960s and the early 1980s were eventful times in Ireland regarding women's and gay rights, contraception and family planning. This mobilisation of people to address these long-standing issues steered to the gay rights movement rather than addressing women's issues, leading to the first Irish responses to HIV/AIDS. Due to the early work of social activists, change was demanded in reproductive rights (McAuliffe and Kennedy 2017), for example, in relation to access to condoms (which was limited only to married couples by prescription) to address the crisis brought by AIDS.

In the early HIV pandemic in Ireland, intravenous drug users were badly affected due to the high levels of HIV within the drug-using community (Foreman and Ni Rathaille 2015). This impacted Irish women in two distinct ways. Firstly, female drug users were the largest Irish group of women with HIV/AIDS during the mid-1980s until the late 1990s (Dorman et al. 1997). Many of these women were from city centre socially deprived areas and at the time, there was a lack of coherent addiction and harm reduction services. Women who used drugs were seen as challenging to deal with and as a social problem from a medical and social perspective due to addiction (Foreman and Ni Rathaille 2015). This lack of visibility of HIV-positive women and mothers in general in the early years of the HIV pandemic in Ireland had a lasting legacy. Additionally, many Irish parents lost adult children to AIDS during the 1980s and 1990s, including people with Haemophilia and gay and bisexual men.

In Ireland, one group of women who were affected by much loss in the early years of the HIV pandemic were the Dublin-based mothers of IV drug users who had died from AIDS. This was during a time when HIV/AIDS was feared and largely believed to be a 'gay disease', rendering it a highly stigmatised illness and many of these women had to grieve privately for their children. Many in society view drug use, in particular injecting opiates, as a high-risk illegal activity and, by association, these women were not afforded much sympathy for their loss. Some of these mothers sought solace in the community arts project, the Irish Names quilt. The AIDS Quilt Project, part of the world's largest community arts project, visually commemorates the life of someone who died from an AIDS-related condition in Ireland by telling their story in a quilt panel (Connell 2020). The quilt was displayed around the country during the Irish AIDS Quilt Group Tour in 1991 and more recently as part of the HIV Ireland 25th anniversary event. It remains an acknowledgement of the loss and impact of AIDS in these communities during the early years of the pandemic.

Having discussed how women were affected during the first couple of decades of HIV/AIDS, we will now move on to a more contemporary review of women with HIV in Ireland in the post-HAART era, where people living with HIV on effective treatment do not have a detectable viral load, meaning it is impossible for them to pass HIV on to anyone else. This is known as U=U (Undetectable = Untransmittable).

7.4 Research of Women and Mothers Living with HIV

In the early years of HIV research, during the 1980s and 1990s, studies with women almost exclusively focused on the prevention of vertical transmission during their pregnancies, in which the health outcomes of foetuses were investigated, but much less so, the health outcomes of their mothers. When pregnant, these women were considered a 'disease' and not a person. The nature of these studies rendered women simply as potential disease vectors from which protection must be sought. As mentioned, the emotional health outcomes of these women (many of whom were newly diagnosed due to antenatal testing) were often not prioritised, illustrating that pregnant mothers living with HIV are seen exclusively as possible threats to their unborn children. Furthermore, women's inclusion in HIV treatment studies was determined based on pregnancy or on their reproductive possibility. This meant that researchers ruled women out of studies to protect unborn and unconceived foetuses, resulting in an unbalanced outcome for gender-specific research and under representation of women in HIV clinical trials (Tariq and Kasadha 2022; Terence Higgin's Trust 2018; DeJong and Battistin 2015; Logie et al. 2012).

Within many societies, women with HIV are viewed as a potential threat to their sexual partners by being positioned as sexually deviant women who do not conform to social sexual norms (Welbourn 2013; Persson 2005; Squire 2003). Consequently, women with HIV were often seen in their capacity as 'vectors of disease', and their position as women with agency was frequently ignored. Faden et al. (1996) originally proposed the concept that WLHIV were constructed as 'vessels and vectors' as biomedical research narrowly focused on women with HIV from the perspective of reproduction and health outcomes on foetuses and pregnancies rather than the health outcomes/wellbeing of the women in the studies. As mentioned, the emotional health outcomes and psychological wellbeing of these women (many of whom were newly diagnosed due to antenatal testing) were often not prioritised in research, highlighting the dominance in which women were viewed through a medical gaze.

Importantly, the researched response to the health needs of infected women can be seen as delayed, considering the first known diagnosis of HIV was in 1981; it was 13 years later, in 1994, before the first major study with women was conducted. Since then, the number of studies with women has increased substantially and has evolved to include women in studies outside of vertical transmission of HIV (Wickremsinhe et al. 2019). However, when women feel forced to conceal their HIV status from others, it can pose a barrier to social support. Many studies have indicated how social support, specifically peer support, can be particularly beneficial in helping women adjust to their diagnosis (Nkosi and Rosenblatt 2019; Paudel and Baral 2015). When women share their diagnosis with others, it often results in support and practical help, which is very beneficial. However, many women avoid telling others, as they anticipate it will result in negative consequences for them, highlighting the social stigma and subsequent shame that many mothers face regarding their HIV status. Therefore, social stigma can affect women's experiences of living with HIV, which can be complicated by their social circumstances, relationships, cultural background, support network and parental responsibilities. Of course, in more recent times, an HIV diagnosis does not have the same consequences that it had before the wide availability of anti-retrovirals and U=U; however, social challenges may persist for many living with HIV.

7.5 Mothering When HIV Positive

Following the birth of their children, many women can feel isolated in the early months. Mothers living with HIV can also experience social isolation compounded by the fact that they may have to deal with poverty, uncertain immigration status, social isolation and intimate partner violence. HIV-positive mothers with newborn babies also need to take steps to prevent vertical transmission in the postnatal period. Indeed, infant feeding can become a concern for these mothers due to the sociocultural meanings of breastfeeding, which are complex and are often class-specific in that not breastfeeding can attract judgement from family and friends.

Tariq et al.'s (2016) UK study explored infant feeding with HIV-positive migrant African mothers, who reported the difficulty of infant feeding decisions from a sociocultural perspective. Importantly, this study found that the availability of safe formula feeding does not necessarily lessen the emotional impact of the decision not to breastfeed. Greene et al.'s (2015) study of Canadian-origin and migrant women living with HIV in Ontario, Canada, also examined this phenomenon within a context of a heavily promoted public health message about the value of breastfeeding as the optimal method of infant feeding. This study highlighted that abstaining from breastfeeding was difficult for mothers as it could unintentionally result in disclosure of an HIV-positive status, as they may have to explain their decision to use formula milk (Greene et al. 2015). These studies thus highlight that not breastfeeding can compromise the maternal well-being of MLHIV.

Despite the increasing normalisation of HIV (Walker 2019; Rodger et al. 2016, 2019b; Beuthin et al. 2015; Moyer and Hardon 2014) due to the success of treatment, the possibility of judgement due to an HIV diagnosis remains a concern for many, including mothers. The advances in the care and treatment of most people living with HIV have lessened the psychosocial impact of being HIV positive, but stigma and discrimination remain part of the HIV experience. For instance, migrant women living with HIV from African countries, where HIV is highly prevalent, may have had previous experiences of the devastation of HIV/AIDS in their home countries. Personal biographies can influence the HIV experience, and studies have shown that migrant African women and mothers sometimes withhold sharing their HIV status from others in an attempt to avoid possible stigma and judgement (Greene et al. 2015).

Currently, in Ireland, most newly diagnosed women are of childbearing age, and often, an HIV diagnosis occurs in early pregnancy due to antenatal testing. For most women, having children is a way to fulfil social roles and identity and is very much an option for HIV-positive women due to the low rate of vertical transmission since the introduction of HAART. Having children when HIV positive brings unique challenges, which include the pregnancy experience, decisions around infant feeding and testing newborns. Being a mother has always been important to women living with HIV; nevertheless, the maternal HIV experience is underrepresented in the literature. Following an HIV diagnosis, the physical, psychological and social consequences of being HIV positive have become more apparent; however, little is known about the mother's experiences post diagnosis, which the next section addresses.

7.6 Gaining an Understanding of MLHIV Experiences

Women who have children either prior to or after their HIV diagnosis face distinct challenges and this next section will draw on research with Irish-based mothers living with HIV (MLHIV). As noted earlier, much research to date with HIV-positive mothers has been situated within the dominant biomedical discourse, focusing more on outcome than on experience. This narrative study aimed to explore the multidimensional impact of maternal HIV infection using a purposive sample of eleven HIV-positive mothers living in Ireland from both high and low-HIV prevalence countries. The participants were at different points on the motherhood trajectory, including mothers of young babies and those with teenagers and adult children. This study included Irish women, African and European women between the ages of mid-20s and early 60s, and two women who were also grandmothers. Most were living with HIV for at least 3 years, and two had been HIV positive for more than two decades. In what follows, selected experiences from this study that shed light on how being HIV-positive affects mothers will be presented. It will present how mothers deal with their HIV diagnosis, the psychosocial experiences of mothering with HIV with specific reference to stigma and the sharing of the diagnosis. This study gives voice to the perspective of the participants and the impact of this diagnosis on their lives.

This study drew on a combination of theoretical standpoints, including HIV stigma frameworks (Campbell et al. 2007; Herek 2002), social capital theory (Putnam 1995), medicalisation and HIV. Narratives are a way to represent and understand significant individual life events (Elliot 2005), as the storytelling process is a collaborative and sense-making process. The use of a narrative approach can be particularly insightful in making sense of and coming to terms with a disruptive health experience like cancer or an HIV diagnosis (Stephens and Breheny 2013).

This study was the first of its kind in Ireland and aims to provide insight into the maternal HIV experience as the women in this study shared stories about their lives. Participants were recruited through an HIV support centre in Ireland. The analysis involved identifying the personal narratives and the collective experience of HIV-positive mothering. This iterative process was to present a synthesis of the commonalities and differences within the narratives, through the use of a narrative analysis framework (Murray 2008). This framework focuses on four specific elements of narratives, which are: the personal, interpersonal, positional and ideological.

This analytical approach allows for greater comprehension of experiences from different perspectives. This highlights differences between women who are mothers and who are often considered a homogeneous group—usually through the medical gaze. Using Murray's narrative framework, what follows will be selected experiences from this study that shed light on how HIV affects mothers. It will present how mothers deal with their HIV diagnosis, the psychosocial challenges of mothering with HIV with specific reference to stigma and the sharing of the diagnosis with others. It will also consider coping strategies used by mothers.

7.7 Becoming an MLHIV

The women in this study shared accounts about both the process of learning about their diagnosis and the ways that they coped with this new and often unexpected information. Some of the women learned about their HIV status as part of their routine antenatal testing, whereas others who were seeking asylum in Ireland had a test as part of their health screening. However, for most women in this study, the diagnosis was unforeseen, as they did not think they were at risk of becoming HIV positive. For example, Suzi, an Irish mother of one son, recounted:

> It was a shock, you know, I was in shock, I could never think, you know, I could get it.

Similarly, Rose, an African woman, upon her diagnosis when pregnant with her third child, said:

> it was a shock, and I was on my own, it was a nightmare, a nightmare.

Both women were not expecting to be HIV positive when diagnosed in the late 2000s. Their surprise diagnosis was due to their belief that they did not fit the profile of those who contract HIV, and so they considered themselves low-risk for HIV. This is not an uncommon reaction.

7.8 Vertical Transmission Worries

Furthermore, mothers and pregnant women newly diagnosed with HIV almost entirely focused on the needs of their unborn/newborn baby, with few speaking about their own personal concerns. For some of the women in this study who had children prior to their diagnosis, they focused on the possibility that their child was also HIV positive but not yet diagnosed. For example, Joanne, who was diagnosed in the mid-1990s shortly after the birth of her son, shared:

> Yes, I was worried until he was eighteen months old 'til I got the all clear, and I was always worried that he'd have it.

Even though the risk of mother-to-child transmission is dependent on the point of infection and older children would not be at risk if their mother had contracted HIV after they were born, testing of children following a mother's diagnosis was an important consideration. Importantly, this may not be information that is widely known due to the lack of awareness and education about the vertical transmission of HIV. Importantly, for most women in this study, whether and when to test their children for HIV, irrespective of the actual risk to their children, affected how they responded to their own HIV-positive result. Significantly, some pregnant women appeared to have an exaggerated sense of the potential of vertical transmission occurring despite being assured by their medical teams that it is preventable, and the likelihood is low. This concern was evident in both newly diagnosed women and those who had been living with HIV for some time, suggesting a unique worry for these mothers. Another issue of grave concern for mothers was the emotional issues associated with the diagnosis, which will now be considered.

7.9 Disclosure: A Challenge for MLHIV

Increasingly, many women do not feel the need to share their HIV status with people around them. The significant medical advancements made in HIV treatment mean that people living with HIV on effective antiretroviral treatment have a normal life expectancy and have the security of knowing they cannot pass it on via unprotected sex if they reach an undetectable viral load (Rodger et al. 2016, 2019a). As a biomedical condition, HIV is now manageable and currently not a threat to one's health; this might influence many women, in which case women may decide not to disclose their HIV status to individuals in their lives. In general, for women, sharing their HIV status can produce beneficial social and peer support, which can contribute to living well with HIV (McLeish and Redshaw 2017; Warren-Jeanpiere et al. 2017; Orza et al. 2015).

However, whether to share one's diagnosis frequently occupies the thoughts of many of those living with HIV (Squire 2012). Some choose not to tell others due to their awareness of the stigma attached to HIV. This can be due to previous knowledge of experiences of HIV-related stigma towards others and an expectation that they, too, will be judged if their status becomes known. So, for pregnant women, their identities as women with HIV are compounded and unique. The nature of HIV being a sexually transmitted virus has contributed widely to its stigmatising discourse (Carter et al. 2017; Welbourn 2013), as well as it being a condition associated with particular groups of individuals, e.g. gay men, intravenous drug use, sex workers. This can translate into concerns for women about how others might perceive their HIV status in light of such stigmatising discourse. Referring back to earlier in the chapter in which we mentioned sexuality and women, the association between sex and HIV can leave these women wondering if they will be devalued as women or mothers after they share their HIV status. This is particularly pertinent for women/mothers navigating friendships and intimate sexual relationships. Keeping one's HIV status concealed may be a protective mechanism from such judgement or disapproval from others. However, it can also prevent women from seeking support to deal with adaptation to life with HIV and the associated psychosocial issues, for example, telling others.

Given the potential for negative reaction to disclosure, it would appear that, in particular for some migrant women, the fear of rejection justified their continued concealment of their HIV status from family and friends. One account from an African migrant woman demonstrates that her continued concealment of her HIV status was due to her belief that she would be judged negatively if it was known. Evelyn's heightened awareness of the relationship between sexual promiscuity and HIV resulted in her reluctance to share it with others. She said:

> They don't know where I got it so they think I am sleeping around and I am not able to explain to them to say, it is my own husband did this to me.

A challenge for mothers relates to an individual's willingness or reluctance to share their diagnosis and the consequences of telling others. A common theme in this research is the additional dilemma of disclosing their HIV status to their children. In this study, participants described that disclosure for them involved how, if and when to tell close friends and their families and sharing their diagnosis with their children. The decision to tell others was affected by the possible consequences of others having this knowledge on their children. Maternal disclosure is unique due to the risk of vertical transmission during pregnancy, and the lack of visibility and general social and cultural lack of knowledge about HIV added to the difficulty women had with telling others. In this study's narratives, participants spoke about their struggle with it because they wanted to protect their children from the burden of HIV for as long as possible. Some in this study had not shared their diagnosis with their adult children and spoke about delaying it for as long as possible. This suggests that they make sense of their non-disclosure by linking it to a desire to protect and to avoid burdening their children. Their assumption that sharing their diagnosis will be detrimental to their children contributes to their reluctance to tell. Notwithstanding that, it can be advantageous to children to know their mother's HIV status as they can be an important source of support. For some women in this study, telling their children was not an option they were willing to consider. Having children also appeared to help the women cope with their HIV and this is a point we will now turn to.

7.10 The Benefits of Being a Mother Living with HIV

In this study, the women acknowledged the value and benefits of motherhood. Developing one's mothering identity and engaging in the duties they associated with mothering generally had a positive impact on their self-perception. For example, Kate shared:

> I'm the same as everybody else now (as a mother), I suppose, as every other woman, I felt so separate before even though there are many women who don't have children but I think the fact that I have had them makes me the same.

Kate found that she was better able to deal with her diagnosis because she felt a bond with other mothers. The benefits of having children were echoed by Elisabeth, who shared:

> For myself, I just told myself that I don't want to think about me being HIV positive. I want to live my life, how can I put it, and not say 'I can't do that because I am HIV positive', so I tend not to think about it, I know I'm going to be there for my kids. I'm going to take my meds and be healthy.

For HIV-positive women with children, it appears their children gave them purpose and determination to manage and deal with the condition and that their identity as mothers was a source of strength to them. Focusing on their maternal responsibilities resulted in a desire to be there for their children by prioritising their needs before considering their own issues. Importantly, the women talked about striving for a sense of normality, as they perceive themselves as 'normal', suggesting that for some, their diagnosis does not define them. This is a positive development for MLHIV and is in tandem with increasing HIV normalisation. As women's experiences of HIV have evolved over the last number of decades, this, in turn, has affected those who have children. From this research, there are some key insights about mothering while HIV positive.

7.11 Conclusion

This chapter foregrounds the maternal HIV experience, which, to date, has received minimal attention with reference to the Irish context. Women's experiences seldom feature in the international and Irish conversations about HIV/AIDS. It drew on a range of historical contexts to inform the contemporary HIV picture as it applies to mothers living with HIV. The second part of the chapter reported some findings from a narrative study with mothers who were HIV positive. It revealed that their HIV diagnosis was unexpected and shocking to them due to their perception that they did not fit the profile of those who become HIV positive. This issue speaks to the lack of relevant information about and for women and mothers living with HIV in Ireland. It is possible that if women are not aware of other women living with HIV, they may not expect that such a diagnosis could happen to them.

The unexpected nature of the diagnosis, in turn, influenced how they responded to their diagnosis, as the lack of readiness can affect one's reaction to the news. Most women unsurprisingly responded in a child-centred way, considering their own health of lesser importance than that of their children. Significantly, this occurs upon diagnosis and cannot be overcome until the HIV status of their children is known; only at that point can mothers look past the 'child-centredness' to consider their own response to the news.

In this study, telling others they had HIV was a concern and included decisions about who needs to know, when to tell them and whether they (the mothers) believed they could cope with the news. These participants were cognisant of the burden that disclosure can place on the recipient and on relationships, despite the ways in which HIV is increasingly a treatable, though chronic condition. This chapter sought to platform knowledge and understanding of women's experiences of HIV, with an emphasis on mothering, as discussed throughout. These issues have often been ignored yet are important in the contribution to stigma eradication.

The study presented contributes to the limited women-centred qualitative studies focusing on mothering with HIV and emphasises that women negotiate many unique challenges as MLHIV. It has scope to inform those who care for them about aspects of their lives that may get little attention during a medical appointment, for example. The inherently gendered experiences highlighted in this chapter remind us how being a mother with HIV is both a biological and social juggling act, even during the increased and accepted HIV normalcy discourses in many countries.

References

Anderson, Jane. 2012. Women and HIV: Motherhood and More. *Current Opinion in Infectious Diseases* 25 (1): 58–65.

Bailey, Linda. 2001. Gender Shows: First-Time Mothers and Embodied Selves. *Gender and Society* 15 (1): 110–129.

Barnes, Donna, Susan Taylor-Brown, and Lori Wiener. 1997. 'I didn't leave y'all on purpose' HIV-Infected Mothers' Videotaped Legacies for Their Children. *Qualitative Sociology* 20: 7–32.

Bennett, David, Kerry Traub, Lauren Mace, Adrienne Juarascio, and Virginia O'Hayer. 2016. Shame Among People Living with HIV: A Literature Review. *AIDS Care* 28 (1): 87–91.

Beuthin, Rosanne, Anne Bruce, and Laurene Sheilds. 2015. Storylines of Aging with HIV: Shifts Towards Sense Making. *Qualitative Health Research* 25 (5): 612–621.

Brion, John, Mark Leary, and Anya Drabkin. 2014. Self-Compassion and Reactions to Serious Illness: The Case of HIV. *Journal of Health Psychology* 19 (2): 218–229.

Bury, Michael R. 1982. Chronic Illness as Biographical Disruption. *Sociology of Health and Illness* 4 (2): 167–182.

Campbell, Catherine, Yogan Nair, Sakhumzi Maimane, and Jonathan Nicholson. 2007. Dying Twice: A Multi-Level Model of the Roots of AIDS Stigma in Two South African Communities. *Journal of Health Psychology* 12 (3): 403–416. https://doi.org/10.1177/1359105307076229.

Carter, A., Greene, S., Money, D. et al. 2017. The Problematization of Sexuality among Women Living with HIV and a New Feminist Approach for Understanding and Enhancing Women's Sexual Lives. *Sex Roles* 77: 779–800.

Connell, Giselle. 2020. Caring for Place with Aids Memorial Quilts in Dublin, Ireland. *Geographical Review* 110 (3): 253–269.

Cuca, Yvette P., and Carol Dawson Rose. 2016. Social Stigma and Childbearing for Women Living with HIV/AIDS. *HIV & Sexual Health* 26 (11): 1508–1511.

Cuca, Y. P., Asher, A., Okonsky, J., Kaihura, A., Dawson-Rose, C., and Webel, A. 2017, Jan-Feb. HIV Stigma and Social Capital in Women Living with HIV. *Journal of the Association of Nurses in AIDS Care* 28 (1): 45–54.

Davtyan, Mariam, Shu Farmer, Brandon Brown, Mojgan Sami, and Toni Frederick. 2016. Women of Color Reflect on HIV-Related Stigma Through PhotoVoice. *Journal of Nurses in AIDS Care* 27: 404–418.

DeJong, Jocelyn, and Francesca Battistin. 2015. Women and HIV: The Urgent Need for More Research and Policy Attention in the Middle East and North African Region. *Journal of the International AIDS Society* 18: 1–3.

Desclaux, Alice, and Marie-Laure Cadart. 2008. Avoir un enfant dans le contexte du VIH: discours médicaux et liens sociaux. *Médecine/Sciences* Special Issue:53–61.

De-Vitri Smith, Sally, Elaine Dietsch, and Ann Bonner. 2013. Pregnancy as Public Property: The Experience of Couples Following Diagnosis of a Foetal Abnormality. *Women Birth* 26 (1): 76–81.

Dorman, A., Keenan, E., Shuttler, C., Merry, J., and O'Connor, J. 1997. HIV Risk Behaviour in Irish Intravenous Drug Users. *Irish Journal of Medical Science* 166 (4): 235–238.

Elliot, Jane. 2005. *Using Narrative in Social Research: Qualitative and Quantitative Approaches.* London: Sage.

Faden, Ruth, Nancy Kass, and Deven McGraw. 1996. Women as Vessels and Vectors: Lessons from the HIV Epidemic. In *Feminism and Bioethics: Beyond Reproduction*, ed. Susan M. Wolf, 252–228. New York: Oxford University Press.

Foreman, Maeve, and Nóirín Ní Rathaille. 2015. Not Just Another Long Term Chronic Illness—Social Work and HIV in Ireland. *Practice.* https://doi.org/10.1080/09503153.2015.1087494.

Greene, Sophie, Adrianne Ion, Dorothy Elston, Gladys Kwaramba, Stephanie Smith, Adriana Carvalhal, and Mona Loutfy. 2015. 'Why Aren't You Breastfeeding?': How Mothers Living With HIV Talk About Infant Feeding in a 'Breast Is Best' World. *Health Care for Women International* 36 (8): 883–901.

Herek, Gregory. 2002. Thinking About AIDS and Stigma: A Psychologist's Perspective. *The Journal of Law, Medicine & Ethics* 30: 594–607.

Hug, Chrystel. 1998. Contraception: From the Protection of Public Morality. In *The Politics of Sexual Morality in Ireland*, ed. Chrystel Hug, 76–108. London: Palgrave Macmillan.

Hutchinson, Phil, and Rageshri Dhairyawan. 2017. Shame and HIV: Strategies for Addressing the Negative Impact Shame Has on Public Health and Diagnosis and Treatment of HIV. *Bioethics* 32: 68–76.

Kelly, Carmen, Fiona Alderdice, Marlene Lohan, and Dale Spence. 2012. Creating Continuity out of the Disruption of a Diagnosis of HIV During Pregnancy. *Journal of Clinical Nursing* 21 (11-12): 1554–1562.

Logan-Kennedy, Victoria, Lena Serghides, Janet Raboud, DeSheng Su, Sandra Blitz, Trevor Hart, and Edward Ralph. 2014. The Importance of Motherhood in HIV-Positive Women of Reproductive Age in Ontario, Canada. *AIDS Care* 26 (6): 777–784.

Logie, Carmen, Llana James, Wangari Tharao, and Mona Loufty. 2012. 'We Don't Exist': A Qualitative Study of Marginalization by HIV-Positive Lesbian, Bisexual, Queer and Transgender Women in Toronto. *Canada, Journal of the International AIDS Society* 15: 1–11.

McAuliffe, Mary, and Sinead Kennedy. 2017. Defending Catholic Ireland. In *Anti-Gender Campaigns in Europe*, ed. Roman Kuhar and David Papernotte, 133–149. London: Rowman Littlefield.

McCarthy, Sarah, J.J. Rasanathan, Anna Crawford-Roberts, Inês Dourado, and Sofia Gruskin. 2014. Contemplating Abortion: HIV-Positive Women's Decision to Terminate Pregnancy. *Culture, Health & Sexuality* 16 (2): 190–201.

McLeish, Jenny, and Maggie Redshaw. 2017. Mothers' Accounts of the Impact on Emotional Wellbeing of Organized Peer Support in Pregnancy and Early Parenthood: A Qualitative Study. *BMC Pregnancy and Childbirth* 17 (28): 1–14.

Moyer, Eileen, and Anita Hardon. 2014. A Disease Unlike and Other? Why HIV Remains Exceptional in the Age of Treatment. *Medical Anthropology* 33: 263–269.

Murray, Michael. 2008. Narrative Psychology. In *Qualitative Psychology: A Practical Guide to Research Methods*, ed. Jonathan A. Smith, 85–101. London: Sage.

Nevedal, Andrea, and Andrea Sankar. 2016. The Significance of Sexuality and Intimacy in the Lives of Older African Americans with HIV/AIDS. *The Gerontologist* 56 (4): 762–771.

Nkosi, Busisiwe, and Paul Rosenblatt. 2019. 'From "Death Sentence to Hope", HIV and AIDS in South Africa': Transforming Shame in Context. In *The Bright Side of Shame*, ed. C.H. Mayer and E. Vanderheiden, 77–87. Cham: Springer.

Nobre, Nuno, Pereira Marco, Roine Risto, Sutinen Jussi, and Sintonen Harri. 2018. HIV-Related Self-Stigma and Health-Related Quality of Life of People Living With HIV in Finland. *Journal of the Association of Nurses in AIDS Care* 29 (2): 254–265.

O'Reilly, Andrea. 2014. *Feminist Mothering*. Albany: State of University of New York.

Orza, Luise, Susan Bewley, Carmen Logie, Elizabeth Tyler Crone, Svetlana Moroz, Sophie Strachan, Marijo Vazquez, and Alice Welbourn. 2015. How Does Living with HIV Impact on Women's Mental Health? Voices from a Global Survey. *Journal of the International AIDS Society* 18 (5): 1–9.

Paudel, Vikas, and Kedar Baral. 2015. Women Living with HIV/AIDS (WLHA), Battling Stigma, Discrimination and Denial and the Role of Supports Groups as a Coping Strategy: A Review of Literature. *Reproductive Health* 12 (53): 1–9.

Persson, Asha. 2005. Women, HIV, and the Heterosexual Encounter. *Presented at The Pozhet Women's Forum, Sydney, November*.

———. 2013. Non/infectious Corporealities: Tensions in the Biomedical Era of 'HIV Normalization'. *Sociology of Health & Illness* 35: 1065–1079.

Proudfoot, Denise. 2014. *A Narrative Exploration of the Experiences of Mothers Living with HIV.* Thesis for Professional Doctorate in Health, University of Bath.

———. 2018. Frozen in a Moment in Time: The Experiences of Mothers Being Diagnosed With HIV Infection. *Journal of the Association of Nurses in Aids Care* 29 (2): 323–329.

Putnam, Robert. 1995. Bowling Alone: America's Declining Social Capital. *Journal of Democracy* 6 (1): 65–78.

Rice, W., Logie, C., Napoles, T., Walcott M., Batchelder, A., Kempf, M. C., Wingood, G., Konkle-Parker, D., Turan, B., Wilson, T., Johnson, M., Weiser, S., and Turan, J. 2018. Perceptions of Intersectional Stigma Among Diverse Women Living with HIV in the United States. *Social Science and Medicine* 208: 9–17.

Rodger, Allison, Valentina Cambiano, and Tina Bruun. 2016. Sexual Activity Without Condoms and Risk of HIV Transmission in Serodifferent Couples When the HIV-Positive Partner Is Using Suppressive Antiretroviral Therapy. *JAMA* 316 (2): 171–181.

Rodger, Allison, Bruun Cambiano Valentina, Vernazza Pietro Tina, Simon Collins, Olaf Degen, Guilio Corbelli, Vicente Estrada, Anna Maria Geretti, Apostolos Beloukas, and Dorthe Raben. 2019a. Risk of HIV Transmission Through Condomless Sex in Gay Couples with Suppressive ART: The PARTNER2 Study Expanded Results in Gay Men. In *22nd International AIDS Conference, Amsterdam.* Abstract WEAX0104LB.

Rodger, Alison, Valentina Cambiano, Tina Bruun, Pietro Vernazza, Simon Collins, Olaf Degen, Giulio Maria, Estrada Corbelli, Geretti Vicente, Anna Maria, Apostolos Beloukas, Dorthe Raben, Pep Coll, Andrea Antinori, Nneka Nwokolo, Armin Rieger, Jan M. Prins, Anders Blaxhult, Rainer Weber, Van Eeden, Brockmeyer Arne, H. Norbert, Amanda Clarke, Del Romero Jorge, Raffi Guerrero, Bogner Francois, R. Johannes, Gilles Wandeler, Jan Gerstoft, Felix Gutiérrez, Kees Brinkman, Maria Kitchen, Lars Ostergaard, Agathe Leon, Matti Ristola, Heiko Jessen, Hans-Jürgen Stellbrink, Andrew N. Phillips, and Jens Lundgren. 2019b. Risk of HIV Transmission through Condomless Sex in Serodifferent Gay Couples with the HIV-positive Partner Taking Suppressive Antiretroviral Therapy (PARTNER): Final Results of a Multicentre, Prospective, Observational Study. *Lancet* 393 (10189): 2428–2438.

Sangaramoorthy, Thurka, Amelia Jamison, and Typhanya Dyer. 2017. Intersectional Stigma Among Midlife and Older Black Women Living with HIV. *Culture, Health and Sexuality* 19 (12): 1329–1343.

Sikstrom, S. 2018. "There was no Love There": Intergenerational HIV Disclosure, and Late Presentation for Antiretroviral Therapy in Northern Malawi. *Social Science & Medicine* 211: 175–182.

Squire, Corinne. 2003. Can a HIV-Positive Woman Find True Love?: Romance in the Stories of Women Living with HIV. *Feminism and Psychology* 13 (1): 73–100.

———. 2012. HIV Disclosure: Practices, Knowledges and Ethics. In *Disclosure in Health and Illness*, ed. M. Davis and L. Masterson. London: Routledge.

Stephens, Christine, and Mary Breheny. 2013. Narrative Analysis in Psychological Research: An Integrated Approach to Interpreting Stories. *Qualitative Research in Psychology* 10 (1): 14–27.

Tariq, Shema, and Bakita Kasadha. 2022. HIV and Women's Health, Where Are We Now? *Women's Health* 18.

Tariq, Shema, Jonathan Elford, Pat Tookey, Jane Anderson, Annemiek de Ruiter, Rebecca O'Connell, and Alexandra Pillen. 2016. 'It Pains Me Because as a Woman You Have to Breastfeed Your Baby': Decision-Making About Infant Feeding Among African Women Living with HIV in the UK. *Sexually Transmitted Infections* 92 (5): 331–336.

Terence Higgin's Trust. 2018. *Women and HIV Invisible No Longer*. London: Terrence Higgin's Trust. http://sophiaforum.net/wp-content/uploads/2018/04/Invisible-No-Longer-full-report-of-a-national-study-of-women-and-HIV.pdf.

Toupin, Isabelle, Kim Engler, Bertrand Lebouché, Joanne Otis, Joseph Lévy, and Myléne Fernet. 2019. Decision-Making About Motherhood Among Women Living with HIV in Canada: A Negotiation of Multidimensional Risk. *Culture, Health & Sexuality* 21 (4): 432–446.

UNAIDS. 2022. *Fact Sheet*. Available at https://www.unaids.org/en/resources/fact-sheet.

Walker, Liz. 2019. 'There's No Pill to Help You Deal with the Guilt and Shame': Contemporary Experiences of HIV in the United Kingdom. *Health* 23 (1): 97–113.

Walsh, Elizabeth, Keith Horvath, Holly Fisher, and Cari Courtenay-Quirk. 2012. The Experiences, Needs, and Internet Use of Women Recently Diagnosed With HIV. *Journal of the Association of Nurses in AIDS Care* 23 (4): 329–338.

Warren-Jeanpiere, Lari, Heather Dillaway, Pilar Hamilton, Mary Young, and Lakshmi Goparaju. 2017. Life Begins at 60: Identifying the Social Support Needs of African American Women Aging with HIV. *Journal of Health Care for the Poor and Underserved* 28 (1): 389–405.

Welbourn, Alice. 2013. Denied Desire: Sexual Pleasure in the Context of HIV. In *Women, Sexuality and the Political Power of Pleasure*, ed. S. Jolly, A. Cornwall, and K. Hawkins, 142–161. London: Zed Books.

Wickremsinhe, Marisha, Margaret Little, Alice Carter, Kristen Sullivan, and Anne Lyerly. 2019. Beyond 'Vessels and Vectors': A Global Review of Registered HIV-Related Clinical Trials with Pregnant Women. *Journal of Women's Health* 28 (1): 93–99.

World Health Organization (WHO). 2024. Global HIV Programme: Mother-to-Child Transmission of HIV. January 02, 2024. https://www.who.int/teams/global-hiv-hepatitis-and-stis-programmes/hiv/prevention/mother-to-child-transmission-of-hiv#:~:text=In%20the%20absence%20of%20intervention, from%2015%25%20to%2045%25.

Zivi, Karen. 2005. Contesting Motherhood in the Age of AIDS: Maternal Ideology in the Debate over Mandatory HIV Testing. *Feminist Studies* 31 (2): 347–374.

Index[1]

[1] Note: Page numbers followed by 'n' refer to notes.

A. Castillo Villanueva, A. Bollas (eds.), *HIV/AIDS in Memory, Culture and Society*, Palgrave Studies in Science and Popular Culture, https://doi.org/10.1007/978-3-031-59699-5

The manufacturer's authorised representative in the EU is Springer Nature Customer Service Centre GmbH, Europaplatz 3, 69115 Heidelberg, Germany. If you have any concerns regarding our products, please contact ProductSafety@springernature.com

Printed and bound by CPI Group (UK) Ltd, Croydon, CR0 4YY
01/10/2026
02225879-0016